Labor of Love

FAMILIES IN FOCUS

Series Editors

Naomi R. Gerstel, University of Massachusetts, Amherst
Karen V. Hansen, Brandeis University
Rosanna Hertz, Wellesley College
Margaret K. Nelson, Middlebury College

Labor of Love

Gestational Surrogacy and the Work of Making Babies

HEATHER JACOBSON

RUTGERS UNIVERSITY PRESS
NEW BRUNSWICK, NEW JERSEY, AND LONDON

Library of Congress Cataloging-in-Publication Data

Jacobson, Heather.
    Labor of love : gestational surrogacy and the work of making babies / Heather Jacobson.
        pages cm. — (Families in focus)
    Includes bibliographical references and index.
    ISBN 978-0-8135-6951-2 (hardcover : alk. paper) — ISBN 978-0-8135-6950-5
(pbk. : alk. paper) — ISBN 978-0-8135-6952-9 (e-book (web pdf))
    1. Surrogate motherhood.   2. Surrogate mothers.   3. Human reproductive
technology—Social aspects.   4. Families.   I. Title.
    HQ759.5.J33   2016
    306.874'3—dc23

                                                                            2015021891

A British Cataloging-in-Publication record for this book is available from the British
Library.

Visit our website: http://rutgerspress.rutgers.edu

Manufactured in the United States of America

For Seiichiro and Miya

Contents

Acknowledgments

This book examines the work of gestating and birthing babies for others and how surrogates[1]—and those around them—understand that labor. My research is based on data I collected through interviewing surrogates; their family members; "intended parents," or those who contract with surrogates; and what I call "surrogacy professionals" (lawyers, physicians, psychologists, surrogacy agency directors, and agency staff members). I thank all of the participants in my study. I am especially grateful to the surrogates, for they have received a fair bit of negative press (something I discuss in this book) and some are therefore reluctant to talk with writers and researchers. Knowing this, I appreciate their willingness to meet with me, to share their stories and introduce me to their families and to their intended parents. My gaining access to the surrogacy community was aided by several surrogacy professionals and surrogates. Though I cannot name them here due to confidentiality, I would like to express my appreciation for their help. I hope this book resonates with surrogates and others in the surrogacy community even if some of my arguments do not reflect their own positions.

During the course of researching and writing this book I enjoyed opportunities to present my work and discuss my research with others. For organizing panels, commenting on my work, or discussing surrogacy and reproductive technologies, I thank Julie Artis, Ann Bell, Peter Conrad, Marianne Cooper, Robin Hognas, Emily Kolker, Annette Lareau, Susan Markens, and Miranda Waggoner. The fabulous fellow members of my writing group, Sarah Damaske and Kristen Shultz Lee, deserve a special bow, for they offered detailed feedback on every chapter.

I thank the editors of the Rutgers University Press's Families in Focus series, especially Peggy Nelson and Karen Hansen, for their insightful discussions about my work, and Rosanna Hertz for her helpful feedback and advice. Peter Mickulas at the press was a supporter of this project from our first discussion early in my data-collection phase. I thank Peter, the reviewers, and the rest of the production staff at Rutgers for their help on this project.

I received assistance from the University of Texas at Arlington (UT Arlington) in the forms of both funding (a Research Enhancement Program grant) and time (a Faculty Development Leave) that enabled me to complete the research on which this book is based. I am grateful for the institutional assistance from UT Arlington and for my colleagues in the Department of Sociology and Anthropology for creating a supportive working environment. Two of my colleagues at UT Arlington, Christian Zlolniski and Amy Speier, deserve special thanks for their extensive comments on my work. I also thank the graduate students in my Sociology of Reproduction and Qualitative Methods classes for our discussions on reproductive technologies and the methods used in this project. Ben Agger deserves special recognition for his support. During the nine years we worked together at UT Arlington, Ben was a true mentor and a wonderful colleague. I will miss him.

The process of researching and writing this book was made more pleasurable because of the support I received from my friends and family. I appreciate the interest my good friend Caroline Florez and my father and stepmother, Ken and Merrilee Jacobson, showed in my work. I thank Nia Parson, Kelly Rayburn, and Nicole Hunter for their friendship and the friendship their families have shown my daughter (allowing Miya some excellent play time with good friends—and me some excellent slices of writing time). My mother, Susan Watt, helped care for Miya and our menagerie of animals, and made innumerable evenings more enjoyable with good food and laughter. I am glad she and my stepfather, Roy Watt, decided to become snowbirds and join us in Texas for part of each year.

My immediate family has lived with this project for a good five years, half the lifetime of my daughter, Miya. This research helped reinforce how much fuller my life is with her in it. I am so grateful for the opportunity to be her mother. My husband, Seiichiro Tanizaki, is my all-hands-on-deck, tell-me-what-you-need pillar of support. Thank you, Seiichiro, for the gift of time you gave me to write this book, your belief in my work, your constancy, and not calling the cops when that one interview took four and a half hours.

Labor of Love

CHAPTER 1

Conceptions

Molly Hughes[1] never imagined it would be so hard to get pregnant. She was a healthy twenty-nine-year-old and had already had two children. With her daughter, Nina, and son, George, she conceived quickly and had enjoyable, uneventful pregnancies and births. When I first met Molly in 2009, she had been trying for three years to get pregnant using advanced reproductive technologies. She had completed four in vitro fertilization (IVF) procedures, none of which had resulted in the birth of a child. Molly was shocked. It had been so easy with her first two pregnancies, and she felt like a failure. In one of the four procedures, the embryo failed to implant. Two other cycles ended in what is known as a "chemical pregnancy," a very early miscarriage in which the embryo does not properly adhere to the uterine wall. Most devastating for Molly, however, was the second trimester miscarriage she suffered. During a routine obstetric exam in her fourteenth week of pregnancy, the technician at Molly's doctor's office could not find a heartbeat. The doctor contemplated having Molly labor and birth the deceased fetus, but instead performed a dilation and evacuation procedure (D&E). Molly was distraught and left to try again with another round of IVF.

As we sat on the couch in her small, tidy East Texas home, Molly let me know that three years of attempting pregnancy was taking a toll on her and on her family. Her husband, Dustin, accompanied her to almost all of her appointments, which were numerous—and many of which were several hours away from their home. Molly was nervous about driving in the big city, and Dustin was there for her—not only as a chauffeur, but also for support. For these visits, Dustin had to take time off work. That was fine, Molly told me, as Dustin was a salaried employee; but still, she said, it "wore on him." Molly, the primary caregiver to their two school-age children, had previously worked in child care and was now looking for part-time work. Sometimes Molly and Dustin would bring Nina and George with them to appointments, but other times, especially when they had to go to the infertility specialist's office (a good four-hour drive away), Molly had to find someone to care for the children. Luckily, she had a good support system in her mother and her best friend. During the previous three years, Molly had been gone from home a lot more than usual due to all of the doctor's appointments. She had to miss some important events in her children's lives—a baseball tournament, a mother and son dance—occasions she would never be able to make up, and she felt bad about that.

Molly's children, Nina and George, had initially been excited by the thought of a baby. But after three years, they had become blasé about the idea that their mom would ever get pregnant. Molly and her doctors, after all, had tried almost everything. Everything, that is, except using Molly's eggs or Dustin's sperm, or creating a child the "old-fashioned way." Molly, you see, had no interest in adding another child to her family; with Nina and George, her family was complete. She was trying to add a child to someone else's family—a family of strangers. For three years, Molly had been trying desperately to succeed as a gestational surrogate.

Gestational Surrogacy

Gestational surrogacy is a relatively new medical procedure, social arrangement, and form of compensated labor in the United States. Gestational surrogates, like Molly, are implanted with embryos via IVF and paid to gestate and bear the resulting children. The people they are helping—the intended parents (IPs)— are unable or in some cases unwilling to get pregnant or carry a pregnancy to term themselves due to infertility, social or medical issues, or because they are men. Though some surrogates undertake altruistic surrogacy and receive no monetary compensation, today most are thought to engage in commercial surrogacy and are paid for their services. At the time I met Molly, however, she had received little compensation for her three years of work. It is only after a successful "journey"—one that ends in the birth of a live baby—that most surrogates receive full compensation.

Though Molly had yet to bring a pregnancy to term, she was not out of pocket; her IPs had paid for all of the medical tests and procedures, office visit copayments, and travel expenses. Her first set of IPs (there had been two sets so far) had compensated her for her three months of pregnancy, according to their contract. Nonetheless, she had invested three years of her life trying to get pregnant for others, people she had not known before meeting them through a surrogacy agency. Why was Molly so intent on being a surrogate? And why did she rearrange her life—and the lives of her family—to do so?

Popular discourse, including the 2008 Tina Fey movie *Baby Mama*, would have us believe that Molly was doing surrogacy solely for the money, that she was "renting her womb" to the highest bidder. Gestational surrogates usually make between $20,000 and $35,000 for successfully completing a journey. But when Molly first started surrogacy, she did not even know that she would get paid. Some surrogates I spoke with even thought at first that they would be responsible for the medical expenses associated with carrying and birthing someone else's child. Not all surrogates, of course, are naive about payment, but the story of surrogacy—including the motivations of women like Molly—is more complicated than a simple cash transaction.

Molly had been working at surrogacy for three years when I first met her. Her life, she told me, had been "consumed by surrogacy." The IVF medical protocol alone was intense. Molly had to take a series of medications—to first regulate her menstrual cycle and then shut it down, to thicken the uterine lining, all to trick her body into thinking it was pregnant so that it would accept a foreign embryo and sustain it. Her husband had to learn how to give her the daily injections, and sometimes they had to forgo outings that coincided with medication timing. She and Dustin had to abstain from sexual intercourse when she was cycling on the medications, especially in the period immediately before and after embryo transfers. Molly wanted to be extremely careful, so she and Dustin had not had intercourse regularly since she began attempting to have a surrogate pregnancy.

For three years, Molly had been on this medical regimen, cycling with nothing to show for it except a deepening understanding of both infertility and the medical reproductive procedures meant to combat it, as well as a lot of heartbreak and frustration. For Molly and her family, those three years had been like a roller-coaster ride. Molly was dedicated, though. She continued to try, and over the course of the next three years she did get pregnant, bearing a singleton for one couple and twins for another. She loved it. She might try again. After six years in the world of surrogacy and seeing the joy on the faces of her IPs, it was hard, Molly told me, to imagine "retiring."

This book examines the experiences of women like Molly who are paid to gestate and bear children for others. The data on which this book is based come from three years spent in the world of surrogacy as a researcher. From the summer of 2009 through the fall of 2012, I interviewed thirty-one surrogates like Molly about their surrogacy journeys and their lives. I also interviewed others intimately involved with surrogacy—IPs, surrogacy agency directors and employees, attorneys, counselors, and psychologists, an infertility doctor, and surrogates' family members and close friends. In all I spoke with sixty-three people about their surrogacy experiences, following many on their journeys through follow-up interviews, e-mail messages, phone calls, and blog updates. I also frequented surrogacy websites, popular online surrogacy forums, and a wide range of surrogacy blogs from 2009 through 2015.

As I spent time in the world of surrogacy, I became more interested in examining surrogacy not from the perspective of IPs and the lens of family formation but, rather, from the perspective of surrogates and the lens of work. I was initially curious, as many are, about the motivations of women who bear children for others. However, I became increasingly fascinated by what I came to realize was quite a complex and laborious process that is largely enacted and often managed by surrogates. This book is the result of that interest, focusing on the work surrogates engage in and how they, and others, understand that labor in a society in which these arrangements have a contentious history.

Surrogacy itself is not a new practice. Those familiar with the biblical story of Abraham, Sarah, and Hagar or the cultural rules of the system of concubines in traditional China know that these arrangements have a long history. In both of those traditions men with infertile wives impregnated women (most often concubines or slaves) to bring children into a marriage. While those traditions are quite old, surrogacy today—particularly its volume, medical options, commercialization, and apparent similarity to paid employment—is rather different.

Contemporary surrogacy was first introduced to many in the United States with the Baby M case of the late 1980s. In that arrangement, the surrogate, Mary Beth Whitehead, contracted with William Stern to conceive via artificial insemination (with Stern's sperm), gestate, and bear the resulting child. The contract stated that Whitehead would relinquish all parental rights and custody, allowing for the child to be adopted by Stern's wife, Elizabeth. Whitehead was to be paid $10,000 and have all of her medical care covered. After the birth of the child, however, Whitehead decided she wanted to parent the baby. There ensued a custody battle and a protracted legal case—all played out before a captivated nation.

Whitehead was what is known as a "traditional surrogate"—that is, one who conceives for others a child who is genetically related to her. In much earlier times, traditional surrogates were the only kind possible, with insemination occurring via sexual intercourse between intended father and surrogate. Today and in Whitehead's case, traditional surrogates conceive via artificial insemination (AI). Beginning in the mid-1970s, AI or traditional surrogacy began to become commercialized, with lawyers and physicians practicing in the field and being compensated for their work, and with some surrogates receiving fees for their time and labor—though not, ostensibly, for their children (Field 1990, 5). It was not until Baby M, however, that many people in the United States became aware that surrogacy was occurring and that a market had developed around these arrangements.

With the exposure that came with the Baby M case, surrogacy and the incorporation of third parties, contracts, and money into birth and parental rights became a political issue and topic of national discussion (Markens 2007). Conservative opponents of surrogacy argue that what they call the natural relationship between husbands and wives, parents and children, and marriage and pregnancy is disrupted with the use of surrogate wombs (E. Roberts 1998).

The Roman Catholic Church, for example, opposes the use of all artificial reproductive technologies and finds the use of surrogates in the creation of children immoral. A 1987 Vatican document presented Catholic objections to surrogacy directly:

> Surrogate motherhood represents an objective failure to meet the obligations of maternal love, of conjugal fidelity and of responsible motherhood; it offends the dignity and the right of the child to be conceived, carried in the womb, brought into the world, and brought up by his own parents; it sets up, to the detriment of families, a division between the physical, psychological, and moral elements which constitute those families. (Congregation for the Doctrine of the Faith 1987)

It is this division between conception, gestation, and parenthood that the Catholic Church and many people find so problematic. Popular cultural conceptions of motherhood in the contemporary United States honor and privilege the unity of biological, gestational, and social mothering. Despite historical and cultural variations in what it means to be a mother, the unity of motherhood today is framed as part of nature itself, with the belief that natural bonding occurs between mother and infant—thanks to their female instinct, women naturally love, understand, and have empathy for and a connection to the children they beget and birth (Glenn 1994; M. Nelson 1990). Surrogacy disrupts that unity by dividing motherhood into distinct activities (donating an egg, gestating and birthing a baby, and parenting that child) and is therefore often seen as an affront to nature (E. Roberts 1998; Teman 2010). In this framework, surrogacy is unnatural because the unity of motherhood and the natural relationship that develops between mother and infant should preclude women from purposefully gestating and bearing children they do not intend to parent, and if they do have such children, it should make it impossible for them to hand those children over to other people.

The introduction of money into these arrangements represented a sea change to some people, who saw it as potentially coercing women, especially poor women, into behaving unnaturally. Commercialized surrogacy is understood to be an extreme example of "the heightened commodification of intimacy that pervades social life" (Boris and Parrenas 2010, 1). As Viviana Zelizer has observed, there is an intense resistance to the overlapping of what are understood as the separate spheres of intimacy and economics; when this does happen, "inevitable contamination and disorder" are thought to result (2005, 20–21; see also 1985). In surrogacy, the argument goes, compensation is understood to push women—especially poor women—to use their bodies unnaturally, as reproductive machines, out of economic desperation (Corea 1985; Oliver 1989). In doing so, women are objectified "by selling their capacity to bear children for a price" (D. Roberts 1997, 277). In an interesting twist that others have noted, on this point of assumed coercion and exploitation Catholic conservatives were in line with a vocal contingent of feminists (Andrews 1989; Macklin 1990; Markens 2007).

Feminist opposition to surrogacy, especially from the 1970s through the early 1990s, focused primarily on the potential commodification of children and the market control of women's bodies that surrogacy allows (see, for example, Corea 1985; Oliver 1989; Rothman 1989). There were also concerns that surrogacy "encourages the point of view that women's primary function is as child-bearers, which reduces women to being 'gestational vessels' with little worth outside reproduction" (Weiss 1992, 16). Unlike conservative opponents, feminists did not (and do not) object to surrogacy on the basis that it threatened the "traditional family"; rather, the issue was the exploitation of women, especially poor women, for their reproductive abilities (D. Roberts 1997; Rothman 1989; Teman 2008).

Though many feminists opposed surrogacy as inherently oppressive to women and stood behind Whitehead, not all felt that surrogacy should be banned. Reproductive autonomy, an important cornerstone of feminist think-ing and activism, was a divisive issue when it came to surrogacy. There were some who argued that reproductive autonomy included the right to participate in surrogacy and that women should have control over their bodies, including the choice to conceive and bear children for others (Andrews 1990; Oliver 1989). Some argued that this right should be exercised but tempered by a ban on paid surrogacy to discourage exploitation (Charo 1990). Others upheld women's rights to engage in contracts and framed as paternalistic conservatives' argument that surrogates cannot fully understand what they are agreeing to: "It questions women's ability to know their own interests and to enter into a contractual arrangement knowingly and competently" (Macklin 1990, 141). This position is visible in the arguments of Lori Andrews, for example, when she imagines possible ramifications of the banning of surrogacy: "Once women are held incompetent to make surrogacy contracts, they may be denied the right to make other contracts. Once policymakers deny women the reproductive choice of surrogacy in order to protect potential children against putative harm, they may deny women other prenatal choices—to undergo amniocentesis or not, to rule out Cesareans, to abort—on those same grounds" (1989, 253). These rights—to make the choice to be a surrogate and to enter into surrogacy contracts—were supported, of course, by surrogacy professionals: surrogacy agency directors and the attorneys and physicians who worked in the field.

Professionals also framed surrogacy in terms of the rights of infertile couples—especially biological fathers (at that time, the surrogates were the bio-logical mothers)—to have children via these traditional surrogacy arrangements (Oliver 1989). This pronatalist right-to-parent discourse has traction in the United States, a country in which parenthood has long been viewed as natural (and "barrenness" as a curse), in which people are pressured to procreate, and

in which investment in our children is very high and seen as not only personally fulfilling but good for the nation (Lovett 2007; Zelizer 1985). It was in 1942,
in *Skinner v. Oklahoma*, that the U.S. Supreme Court framed "marriage and
procreation [as] fundamental to the very existence of the survival of the race"
and "one of the basic civil rights of man."[2] The *Skinner* case was challenging the
compulsory sterilization of criminals (Cahn 2009; D. Roberts 1997), and with
the development of advanced reproductive technologies, this "basic civil right"
to procreate became complicated in ways that the Supreme Court might not
have imagined in 1942.

Notions of the right to a family in the contemporary United States and what
constitutes family, especially the child-parent relationship, rely heavily on the
connections that are thought to derive from genetic linkages between people
(Jacobson 2008). This shapes who are seen as family members and supports the
notion that one's "real children" are only those who arrived through the biological route to parenthood (Wegar 1997). Of course, this notion is not held by all
and is challenged by many people, including those in adoptive families, stepfam-
ilies, blended families, foster families, and families that have used egg or sperm
donation and surrogacy. As others have argued, however, in addition to the ways
assisted reproductive technologies challenge notions of the "traditional family,"
they also reinforce them and privilege biological parenthood. This can be seen
in the way that surrogate professionals justify their practices by presenting the
need for biological children and the right to have what they call "real children"
of "one's own," to "pass on one's genes," as a natural desire of all people, one the
professionals do not create or shape but are only attempting to help people fulfill.
This "right" is also articulated by the consumers of reproductive technologies,
who come to see reproduction as a basic human right (Becker 2000).

Feminists have long critiqued pronatalism and the pressure women—
especially white, middle-class women—historically have experienced to procreate (Lovett 2007; D. Roberts 1997). Under pronatalism, being a "good woman"
in the United States is equated with motherhood, establishing a "motherhood mandate" that coerces or forces women to mother and to think about
themselves primarily as mothers (Glenn 1994; Russo 1976). However, the
motherhood mandate has social class and racial dimensions, with working-
class or poor women and women of color more challenged in fulfilling the
middle-class ideal of proper mothering (that is, intensive and full time) (Hays
1996; McCormack 2005). Scholars have shown important ways in which the
reproductive capacity of women of color and poor women is, and historically
has been, policed, while reproduction is encouraged among the white middle
class (Cahn 2009; Lovett 2007; D. Roberts 1997). For example, the eugenics
movement, which began in the United States at the beginning of the twentieth
century, promoted "reproductive strategies that would ensure higher rates of
reproduction among the fit [read: middle-class whites] and lower rates among

the unfit [read: poor women and women of color]" (Solinger 2005, 89). Some argue that this schism between encouraging and policing reproduction has intensified with the development of new reproductive technologies, denying poor women of color alternative reproductive possibilities while encouraging middle-class women to devote more time, energy, and money in attempting biological motherhood (Becker 2000; Bell 2014). Opponents of assisted reproductive technologies also "object to the naive technological optimism inherent in the mainstream view [that these technologies are inherently good] and raise questions about who will control the new technologies"—and for what purpose (Purdy 1996, 75). They are concerned about the ways in which the existence of the technologies and how they are used "reinforce harmful biologically determinist stereotypes of women" (ibid., 76).

Surrogacy is seen by some as coercive pronatalism that encourages surrogates to find their worth in their reproductive capabilities while at the same time stripping them of their maternal rights. For example, Barbara Katz Rothman, a leading feminist opponent of surrogacy, writes that she is "horrified" by surrogacy because it "reinvents motherhood." "If any pregnant woman," she continues, "is not necessarily, inherently, legally, morally, and obviously the mother of the baby in her belly, then no woman can stand firm before law and the state in her motherhood" (2011, 202). There is something unique, this argument posits, about the relationship between a woman and the fetus she is gestating—even if she is not the genetic mother. We have enshrouded that position in a social relationship (mother) and given it legal status (also mother). This framing positions surrogacy as particularly problematic because it allows the pregnant woman to be downgraded or completely obscured and the focus purely to be placed on the product: the baby. This is a dangerous precedent with potential legal complications for all mothers, Rothman and others contend (D. Roberts 1997). For example, the obscuring of the pregnant woman via surrogacy is in step with the political and medical movement to treat the fetus as a person, which has been used in the anti-abortion campaign (Hartouni 1997).

It was this exact issue, the legal relationship between mother and child, that was the focus of the Baby M case. Whitehead was being asked to rescind her rights to her biological child, against her will, to comply with the contract she had freely signed prior to conceiving the child. The court was ruling on whether or not Whitehead could be contractually obliged to relinquish her parental rights. A lower court ruled that she could be required to do so, finding that "the constitutional privacy rights of childless couples demand state validation and specific enforcement of surrogacy agreements" (Allen 1988, 1). With this finding, custody was given to William Stern and Whitehead's parental rights were terminated, enabling Elizabeth Stern to adopt the child. This finding was overturned less than a year later by the New Jersey Supreme Court, and Elizabeth Stern's adoption of the child was invalidated. The court ruled that the surrogacy contract could not be enforced, but rather the custody of the child needed to be determined based on the child's best interests.

The case of Baby M, therefore, was "transformed . . . from a contract dispute into a custody proceeding" and largely evolved (some would say devolved) into character judgments about the Sterns and the Whiteheads and the question of which set of parents would be best for the child (Cahn 2009, 101). The New Jersey Supreme Court ruled that the surrogacy contract was void. The question remaining was: Who should have the child? Experts were brought in to evaluate Whitehead's fitness as a mother. They found her lacking (though many found the experts themselves lacking). The deck, some argue, was stacked against her. Whitehead was described in the press as a high school dropout who "married at 16, [and] had two children before she turned 19" with her husband, an "episodic alcoholic" sanitation worker ("Who's Who in the Fight for Baby M" 1987; see also Myers 1989). The Sterns, on the other hand, were middle-class professionals: she a pediatrician, he a biochemist. His family had perished in the Holocaust. She had a mild form of multiple sclerosis (which had made them decide to use a surrogate). Much was made in the press of the class differences between the two couples. According to opinion polls conducted at the time, the general public supported the Sterns as parents for the baby (Markens 2007, 22). The New Jersey Supreme Court agreed, awarding custody to William Stern, though Whitehead retained her status as legal mother and was given visitation rights.[3]

The issues raised in the Baby M case have played a large role in shaping understandings of surrogacy and, as I argue in this book, contemporary surrogacy practices. That case is, therefore, a good place to begin thinking about the contemporary surrogacy market, what we know (or think we know) about surrogacy, and what the issues regarding these arrangements are today.

Much of the academic work on surrogacy arose around this famous case (see, for example, several edited volumes dedicated to the case such as Bartels et al. 1990 and Gostin 1990). Scholarship on surrogacy has primarily been either psychological in nature, focusing on surrogates' motivations, or political in nature, focusing on the ethical quandaries involved, including those related to the coercive forces that propel women to engage in surrogacy (see, for example, Andrews 1989; Anleu 1992; Braverman and Corson 1992; Ciccarelli and Beckman 2005; Corea 1985; Edelmann 2004; Field 1990; Hanafin 1984; Ketchum 1992; Lane 2003; Macklin 1990; Oliver 1989; Purdy 1996; E. Roberts 1998; Teman 2008; van den Akker 2007). There have also been policy-oriented studies on surrogacy and examinations of surrogacy legislation in the United States and abroad (see, for example, Charo 1990; Field 1990; Franklin 1993; E. Nelson 2013; Rao 2003). For example, Susan Markens (2007), in her analysis of the legislative responses to surrogacy in New York and California, shows how social and cultural factors shaped the early public debates on surrogacy in the 1980s and 1990s. Collectively, this rich scholarship on surrogacy is embedded in a much larger literature on the legal, social, and ethical issues related to assisted reproductive technologies and changing alternatives for family formation (see, for example, Becker 2000; Cahn 2009, 2013; Ettorre 2002; Franklin 1995; Hartouni 1997; Purdy 1996; D. Roberts 1997; Rothman 1989; Shanley 2001; Solinger 2005; Spar 2006; Thompson 2005).

Interestingly, however, though there has been recent ethnographic scholarship on surrogacy in other places around the globe, such as Israel (Teman 2010) and especially India (DasGupta and Das Dasgupta 2014b; Hochschild 2012; Nayak 2014; Pande 2008, 2009, 2010a, 2010b, and 2014; Rudrappa 2010 and 2012), there has been little empirical research detailing the processes, relationships, and structure of surrogacy in the United States—the world epicenter of surrogacy. Only a handful of studies by social scientists have examined the lived experience of surrogacy in the United States. Through in-depth interviews with participants in surrogacy, Elizabeth Roberts (1998) analyzed the ways surrogates subvert surrogacy discourse that treats them as unnatural. Centering on the relationship between a single surrogate and her intended mother, Gillian Goslinga-Roy (1998 and 2000) explored the concept of agency and the embodied surrogacy experience via interviews and the production of an ethnographic film. Zsuzsa Berend (2012) examined surrogate mothers' online discussions, finding that the relationship between surrogates and intended mothers was central to the surrogacy experience. However, Helena Ragone's *Surrogate Motherhood: Conception in the Heart* (1994) is the only published large-scale interview-based ethnography of surrogacy in the United States. This is surprising, as surrogacy is largely a US phenomenon; most other advanced countries have outlawed the practice. Much of what we know about surrogacy in the United States comes from Ragone's pathbreaking work. Ragone contextualized the public debate raging on surrogacy and gave a face and a voice to women engaged in surrogacy arrangements. Her ethnography illuminated the ways women negotiate the complex terrain of "traditional motherhood" where it intersects with third-party pregnancy.

Ragone's research, like the majority of the existing scholarship, focuses largely on traditional, not gestational, surrogacy and is based on data from the late 1980s and early 1990s. Both the organization and experience of surrogacy at that time were qualitatively different from what they are today. Commercial surrogacy was relatively new then: there were few surrogacy agencies, few births, and even fewer surrogates—the overwhelming majority of whom engaged in surrogacy only once, and many of whom did so without compensation. One of my motivations for pursing this research, therefore, was a feeling that although surrogacy is a growing trend that many people have strong opinions about, our grasp of surrogacy in the United States is limited due to a lack of up-to-date ethnographically informed research on the subject.

Although surrogacy has changed so much today from the late 1980s, the concerns raised in Baby M case remain. The debate on surrogacy continues, and consensus is far off. There is still no federal regulation or monitoring of surrogacy arrangements in the United States. State positions on and regulations of the practice vary widely and shift continually. Some states have statutes permitting surrogacy, while others criminalize the practice (Hinson and McBrien 2011). However, these positions change frequently, which points to the continuing larger cultural debate about whether surrogacy (paid or unpaid, traditional or gestational) should exist at all. This debate is larger than the singular case of Baby M and who should have custody of children resulting from surrogacies. It is entrenched in a broader cultural battle over the meaning of motherhood and the relationships between women and the children they bear, on the one hand, and the family, market, and state, on the other hand.

In some ways, things are even more complicated today than they were with Baby M. With traditional surrogacy, especially arrangements made for heterosexual married couples, the lines are clear: a birth mother conceives a child, her biological child, via artificial insemination using the sperm of the intended father. She rescinds her parental rights (often today through a prebirth order), and the wife of the biological father (if he is married) adopts the child. If the arrangement goes smoothly (and most do), this transfer of the mother's rights looks an awful lot like traditional second-parent adoption. Today, however, with gestational arrangements, medical technologies have advanced so much that it is possible to have an embryo created using the gametes of IPs or of sperm and egg donors (that IPs have purchased), grown for several days in a laboratory, frozen for months or years, thawed, and then implanted in a surrogate. After delivery, the child can then be raised by the IPs who coordinated (and paid for) her creation and birth.

When the surrogate is no longer the biological mother, but a third party, an important member of a "reproductive team," the dilemma of biology—of a surrogate "giving up" "her" child—is removed. Socially and in some states legally, this makes for a much simpler expression of parental status and transfer of parental rights. This is an extremely attractive feature for the three main groups of surrogacy players—the IPs, the surrogates, and the surrogacy professionals (American Society for Reproductive Medicine 2012c; Parente 2004). This greater simplicity, coupled with improved success rates, has resulted in an increase in the number of surrogacies. It is difficult to capture accurate rates of surrogacy as there is no official tabulation, but estimates (extrapolated to 2015, based on my calculations) range from ten thousand to thirty-one thousand paid surrogate births in the United States since the late 1970s (Organization of Parents through Surrogacy n.d.; Teman 2010). Today, gestational surrogacy is understood to account for the majority of the estimated 1,500 surrogate births per year (American Society for Reproductive Medicine 2012c; Kleinpeter 2002; Markens 2007; Shanley 2001; Teman 2010).

In other ways, however, gestational surrogacy involves much more complex questions—in social, legal, and philosophical terms—than traditional surrogacy does: When the surrogate is no longer the biological mother, who exactly is she? When biological motherhood and physical gestation are separated and when gestation and birthing are monetarily compensated, how do we make sense of the connection between the woman and the child? In many ways, our medical technologies have outstripped our cultural understandings and outpaced our laws and abilities to regulate these new practices.

Contemporary surrogacy is particularly complicated when we consider compensation. When gestational surrogates are paid—and most of them are today—for their time and suffering, are they workers, employees of the IPs or of the surrogacy agencies? When women engage in surrogacy multiple times is that employment? How do surrogates experience and conceptualize their labor and their related compensation? How does Molly Hughes, for example, understand her six years as a gestational surrogate, and what can that tell us about the contemporary state of work, family, and reproduction? These questions became clear to me when I entered the field and began interviewing surrogates. As I sat with Molly and other surrogates in their homes and listened to their surrogacy journeys, as I watched videos of births and looked through planners of their surrogacy-related appointments, I was impressed by the amount of work they engage in and their dedication to it. However, when I began to delicately approach the topic of surrogacy as work, I met resistance. This came from surrogacy professionals, from surrogates' husbands and adult children, and most strongly from surrogates themselves. I quickly learned that while my understanding of surrogacy as labor was not meant as condemnation of these arrangements, there was something particularly egregious about articulating the idea that surrogacy was work to those involved.

Like Molly, however, many surrogates told me that their surrogate work was "all-encompassing" in that surrogacy "takes over" their lives. It is clearly more than a casual hobby. It becomes part of their everyday routine, with many hours, days, weeks, months, and years required to complete the necessary tasks and related activities. Some of the women in my study had been surrogates for more than a decade, helping three, four, or even five couples bring children into their families. Surrogacy becomes a deep part of their identity: they are surromoms, with their IPs and surro-babies, on surrogacy journeys. Yet they are not—or do not want others to think they are—workers. Why? Surrogacy in the United States at the beginning of the twenty-first century involves not only pregnancy but also medically complicated procedures and somewhat tricky social dynamics, often coupled with a complex burden of work-family balance, that are largely managed by surrogates themselves. They work. And they value the work they do. Yet, as the following chapters show, that work is often hidden from public view, from popular understandings, and even from acknowledgment within the world of surrogacy itself. *Labor of Love* asks why that is so. Why is the work of surrogacy largely obscured?

To answer this question, I argue that we must look at the way surrogacy taps into deep social and cultural understandings of the family and how we as a society seek to protect the notion that our children and our families in general are separate from the market. *Labor of Love* examines those understandings as it explores the everyday work and family experiences of commercial gestational surrogates. In the following chapters, I examine the history of surrogacy in the United States as I explain the contemporary gestational surrogacy market. The motivations of surrogates are described as I examine how surrogates negotiate the complex ideological discourse of work and family within the reproductive marketplace. I then explore the different relationships that develop in the world of surrogacy—relationships between surrogates and their agencies, between surrogates and their IPS, and between IP families and surrogates' families. I also consider how surrogates' conceptions of themselves, reproduction, and birth shift through their relationships with IPs and their experiences in the world of surrogacy. Throughout the book, I explore why there is a strong resistance to thinking about and talking about surrogacy as work, and I give empirical evidence of how the obscuring of surrogacy labor—by the marketplace, surrogacy professionals, IPs, surrogates' families, and surrogates themselves—takes place. In doing so, *Labor of Love* not only documents this new form of work and producing children, but it also aims to help us understand what gestational surrogacy means for surrogates and their families, for the intended parents, and, ultimately, for the rest of us.

CHAPTER 2

Making Reproduction Profitable

THE CONTEMPORARY
SURROGACY MARKET

Patricia Emerson and her husband, Matthew, decided they would wait to have children until they were in their early thirties and established in their careers. Married in her midtwenties, Patricia checked with her doctor first to make sure it was okay to wait. Patricia and Matthew knew they wanted to have children and wanted to have a responsible plan in place. Patricia's obstetrician-gynecologist (OB/GYN) assured her that waiting was not a problem, saying that many of his patients had children in their early thirties. He gave Patricia his blessing, so to speak, and, as each year progressed, a clean bill of health.

When she was thirty, Patricia went to see her primary care physician as she had been feeling excessively tired. The physician took one look at her and ordered blood work. When the results came in the next day, he called her into the hospital for a blood transfusion. "I don't know how you are standing," he told her. It turned out that Patricia had a fibroid tumor condition that was causing her to lose too much blood with each menstrual cycle. She was, according to her physician, literally "bleeding to death."

Her new OB/GYN—she did not return to the one who had given her a clean bill of health only three months before her transfusion—removed a hundred fibroid tumors from her uterus. He also wanted to perform a hysterectomy, but Patricia did not consent to that. She desperately wanted to have a child, having waited and planned for parenthood along with her husband for years. "The only way you give me a hysterectomy," Patricia told the OB/GYN, "is if I am dying. Otherwise, you do everything you can to save my uterus."

Due to their desire to have a child, Patricia and Matthew sought out a reproductive endocrinologist (RE), as they knew that Patricia's medical condition and surgeries would make it improbable that they could achieve pregnancy on their own. REs, surgical subspecialists in obstetrics and gynecology, work with patients experiencing infertility. Patricia's RE thought that she might be able to get pregnant and agreed to perform surgery to "clean up" her uterus to try to develop a uterine lining conducive to pregnancy. Following the surgery, however, the RE told Patricia that he had never seen anything like her uterus: only fatty tissue had grown back; the rest was just scar tissue. There was absolutely no chance for her to carry a child. "I won't even attempt to get you pregnant," he said. However, he went on to tell her in a very positive way: "That's the bad news. The good news is you can have a baby. Your ovaries are completely intact, and all we have to do is put you through IVF [in vitro fertilization] and extract the eggs, and then take your husband's sperm and create embryos. So we just need to get you a surrogate."

"We just need to get you a surrogate"—the phrase puzzled Patricia. At that point, she told me, "I had no idea about surrogacy. Just from the few Lifetime movies I've seen, that's my only exposure to surrogacy. So I'm thinking to myself, 'How am I ever going to find a surrogate?' I'm nervous, and I'm very upset." Her RE, however, told her not to worry, "it's going to be fine." And it was. After several false starts, she found a surrogate in a streamlined and supportive process via a local surrogacy agency. When we first spoke, embryos had been created using Patricia's eggs and her husband's sperm and transferred into the surrogate. Several years later, Patricia now has two children, both born via surrogates.

The ease with which Patricia's RE suggested surrogacy, the confidence he had in surrogate arrangements, and the fact that Patricia went in the course of several years from total inability to carry a child to mothering her genetic children are testaments to advanced medical practices and the institutionalized structure of surrogacy today. Had Patricia experienced a similar medical issue twenty-five years ago, her physician might have suggested traditional surrogacy, in which the surrogate is artificially inseminated and is, therefore, the genetic mother. Most likely, however, he would have suggested adoption as a route to motherhood for Patricia. In the second decade of the twenty-first century, however, gestational surrogacy, allowing both intended fathers and mothers genetic parenthood, is an increasingly popular route to family expansion for those experiencing infertility.

This chapter examines how surrogacy came to be an option for women like Patricia who desire children but are unable to conceive and carry a pregnancy, and who now have the possibility of genetic parenthood via gestational arrangements. In examining the history of surrogacy in this chapter, I look particularly at the surrogacy market—at the structure, players, rules, and discourse—and how it shapes who participates as intended parents (IPs) and as surrogates in this new route to parenthood.

THE EMERGENCE OF A COMMERCIAL SURROGACY MARKET

The commercial surrogacy market is a relatively recent phenomenon. It is predicated on two marketed medical developments: artificial insemination and in vitro fertilization (IVF). As explained in the previous chapter, the surrogacy market first began to develop around traditional surrogacy—arrangements in which women, like Mary Beth Whitehead from the Baby M case, were artificially inseminated with the intended father's sperm and conceived and bore children using their own eggs. The surrogate would then release her parental rights, and, if the IPs were a heterosexual married couple (which they are thought to have been in the majority of early surrogacy arrangements), the intended mother would adopt the child.

Artificial insemination has existed since the 1700s, and donated sperm have been regularly used by women with sterile husbands for over a century, but a medical market for sperm and artificial insemination procedures did not take off until the 1970s (Almeling 2011, 4; Corea, 1985, 310; Field 1990; M. Nelson, Hertz, and Kramer 2013; D. Roberts 1997, 283). With that new market, it was mostly attorneys such as Noel Keane in Michigan, but also some physicians, who saw an opportunity to broker surrogacy contracts. They placed ads in newspapers asking women to "help an infertile couple." These new brokers, hired by IPs, found women to act as surrogates, wrote the contracts, and generally oversaw the process, but it really was uncharted territory. The field of surrogacy in the late 1970s and early 1980s, if it could even be called that, has been described as "fly-by-night" and "piecemeal" (Spar 2006, 71; see also Annas 1990). It was unstructured and had not yet been institutionalized. In other words, any rules that existed were very loose, and any structure was ad hoc. Sometimes surrogates were paid for their services, but sometimes they had only their medical expenses covered. Sometimes surrogates and IPs interacted frequently throughout the process, but sometimes there was virtually no interaction between the parties (Ragone 1994). Most women who acted as surrogates did so only once, and there were very few of them—perhaps only a hundred by 1981 (Field 1990, 5; Spar 2006, 82). This emerging market was small; in the early years there were only a few surrogacy brokers in operation. A true surrogacy market and a true surrogate labor force had not yet solidified.

The emerging surrogacy market was possible due to the fact that reproductive medicine is undergirded by neoliberalism—unregulated free-market capitalism—in the United States (Almeling 2011). Whereas other countries, such as the United Kingdom and Australia, have strong government regulation of reproductive technologies and legislation that outlaws compensated surrogacy, in the United States there is an open market and free trade. And what a market it is! Infertility, which is thought to affect "about 12% of the [US] reproductive-aged population," generates an estimated $3 billion annually (American Society for Reproductive Medicine 2010, 4; see also Spar 2006, 3).

There is no federal regulation or monitoring of surrogacy in the United States. Three government agencies do monitor and collect data on the medical procedures, laboratory testing, drugs, and devices used in assisted reproductive technologies (ARTs), including the screening and testing of sperm: the Centers for Disease Control and Prevention (CDC), the Food and Drug Administration, and the Centers for Medicare and Medicaid Services (American Society for Reproductive Medicine 2010). However, none of these agencies regulates or monitors surrogacy per se. There are professional medical associations, such as the American Society for Reproductive Medicine and the Society for Assisted Reproductive Technology (SART), that issue guidelines for practitioners of assisted reproduction and surrogacy. These are only guidelines, however, and compliance with them is totally voluntary (Hochschild 2012). There are no federal regulations for surrogacy procedures, practices, or fee structures.

Debora Spar argues that the reluctance of the federal government to impose any limits on "the baby business," such a revenue-rich industry, is a reflection not only of "a typical laissez-faire response to emerging markets" but also of "a profound fear of religious or ethical entanglement" (2006, 228). This is especially apparent in surrogacy, which raises questions with a history of contentious ethical and religious debate in the United States, questions regarding procreative liberty, parentage, and parental rights, such as: Who has the legal rights to a developing fetus? Who is the legal mother of that fetus and of the child, once she is born—the woman gestating her, who has no genetic link to her and makes no claim to her, or the one from whose egg she was created and who plans to raise her? What if an egg donor is used—who is the mother then? Who has the right to make decisions regarding the pregnancy—especially decisions that are highly contentious, ethical, and religious, such as those regarding prenatal testing, selective reduction of multiple embryos, and termination? The federal government has thus far avoided any direct discussion of surrogacy that would answer these types of questions on the federal level.

The strong neoliberal orientation that dominates in the United States, coupled with the fact that the federal government remains mute on the topic, makes the United States unique in the world in having so many forms of surrogacy, configurations of donation, and fee structures available—if not in one state, then in another. The United States has, therefore, become a destination for reproductive tourism (E. Nelson 2013). Intended parents from around the globe—especially countries in which compensated surrogacy is illegal, such as Australia, Canada, France, Italy, and the United Kingdom—seek the services of surrogate agencies, REs, and surrogates in the United States. Some IPs, including some from the United States, also travel to other countries such as India and Mexico, where surrogacy fees are cheaper than in the United States. Many Americans who travel abroad for reproductive services do so only after they have been priced out of the US market (Speier 2011). So while surrogacy is a global market, its epicenter remains the United States.

The women who contracted as surrogate mothers in the 1970s, the 1980s, and into the early 1990s were largely bearing their own genetic children.[1] Because of this, their arrangements resembled traditional adoption, and many members of the legal community approached the arrangements as if these were adoptive situations. Adoption was a known legal quantity; surrogacy was not. Adoption was used as the legal model for surrogacy because initially there were no state laws, regulations, or litigation precedents governing surrogate arrangements. In the early years, therefore, surrogates were conceptualized legally as birth mothers (genetic birthing mothers) who relinquished their parental rights after birth (unlike intended fathers, who were the genetic parents, intended mothers in early traditional surrogacy had no independent legal rights to the children until adoption proceedings were concluded after birth).

Those in the world of surrogacy resisted this adoption framing from the outset, arguing that because the children were created with the intent of surrogacy, these cases were fundamentally different from adoptive situations. Intent was an important concept from the beginning of third-party reproduction, and it remains so today. Unlike birth mothers in adoption situations, surrogates do not accidentally find themselves pregnant and then make adoption plans for their child. Rather, these children are created from the outset with the intent of being raised by someone other than the gestating woman. In the surrogacy culture, therefore, these children are viewed as the IPs' child, even if the surrogate is the genetic mother. Despite this discourse of intent, traditional surrogacy in the early years involved a transfer of maternal rights after birth. Legally, this was adoption.

The degree to which this legal adoption framing was problematic for surrogacy depended on the state in which surrogates gave birth (not the state in which the IPs resided). Adoptions in the United States are regulated at the state level; surrogacy followed suit. Traditional surrogacy was challenging, therefore, in states that restricted adoption proceedings through forbidding compensation in adoption arrangements or prohibited the preplacement of children (when birth parents consent before birth "to the adoption of their child by an unrelated, prospective adoptive parent" [State of Michigan Department of Human Services n.d.]).[2] Although all states forbid baby selling, some allow compensation to birth mothers (for medical expenses or rent, for example) while others forbid it, seeing it as payment for babies (Ademec and Miller 2007; Holder 1990).[3] This was a problem for those pioneering attorneys who were brokering traditional arrangements, as surrogacy involves the preplacement of children and, often, compensation.[4]

During the 1980s, several states developed positions specifically about surrogacy, but only fifteen states had any laws or statutes on the books about surrogacy by 1992—most states remained (and many continue to remain) mute on the topic (Andrews 1992; Markens 2007). As of this writing, twenty states have no case law or statutes on surrogacy. Surrogacy takes place in those states as there is no law to prohibit it, but the legality of the arrangements has not been tested.

Of the states that do have statutes or case law, most are supportive of surrogacy. Only three states—New York, Michigan, and Washington—and the District of Columbia have imposed criminal penalties for contracted, compensated surrogacy.[5] Surrogacy is restricted in New Jersey due to case law (the case of Baby M).[6] Three other states (Arizona, Indiana, and Nebraska) have declared gestational surrogacy contracts void and unenforceable but do not impose criminal penalties. In twenty-three other states some form of compensated surrogacy is currently permitted by state statute or supported by case law. However, few states have statutes that permit gestational surrogacy arrangements, regulate those arrangements, and, importantly, enforce surrogacy contracts (Creative Family Connections n.d.). Among the surrogacy friendly states are California and Texas, the two states in which I gathered data for this book.[7]

The surrogacy-friendly legislation in California and Texas gives IPs not only legal procedures for getting their names on birth certificates but also legal protection should enforcement of the contact be necessary.[8] The enforcement of surrogacy in these two states is not without limitation: certain restrictions must be followed to qualify for state protection (Creative Family Connections n.d.). Both states require surrogacy contracts to be filed in state court prior to embryo transfer and cover only gestational arrangements, not traditional ones (Legislative Counsel of California n.d.; Texas Family Code n.d.). In Texas the IPs must be in a legally recognized marriage with each other, which has excluded those in same-sex partnerships since only heterosexual marriage has been recognized by the state of Texas (Texas Family Code n.d.).[9]

When state criteria are met and proper procedures followed, IPs in these two states can have their parental status legally confirmed before a child is born and can have their contracts enforced should any problems arise. IPs who do not meet their state's requirements can have a prebirth order issued, but they are not guaranteed to get one—that depends on their having a good attorney, a sympathetic judge, and a strong case. This is true in many states except for those that have explicit restrictions on surrogacy.

It is the issue of state enforcement that has been central to the surrogacy debate and a key concern of all surrogacy parties (surrogates, IPs, and brokers) since the 1970s. Can the state force women to comply with surrogacy contracts they no longer wish to honor? Can IPs be forced to assume legal guardianship for a child resulting from a pregnancy they had wanted to abort but could not because the surrogate refused the procedure? Can surrogates be forced to have abortions or prenatal testing (such as amniocentesis) or to undergo selective reduction? Many surrogacy arrangements take place in a legal limbo in which these questions cannot be answered because there are no statutes or case law in the states in which they take place; there are statutes, but they have no provisions for enforcement and thus no teeth; or there are strong state statutes or case law, but the IPs are not eligible for protection. Many people engaged in surrogacy, therefore, attempt to fly under the radar, with all parties hoping and trusting that everything will go smoothly, they will be assigned a sympathetic judge who will issue a prebirth order, and no one will change his or her mind.

It is often this type of surrogacy, occurring in states where there is nothing on the books or no protection for surrogacy, that results in litigation and draws public interest. This was the situation with Baby M and more recent cases—such as one in 2007 involving a Florida traditional surrogate, Stephanie Eckard, who decided to parent the child after she had a falling out with her IP couple, or the 2013 case involving a Connecticut gestational surrogate, Crystal Kelley, who fled to Michigan (where she would be declared the legal mother) when she and her IPs fought over whether or not to abort the abnormally developing fetus (Celizic 2007; Cohen 2013).

It is impossible to know exactly how many surrogacy arrangements have gone awry as there is no federal monitoring or data collection—let alone regulation—of these proceedings. Enforcement was particularly shaky and contentious in the early years, when most surrogates were the genetic mothers of the children, simply because there were no state statutes or legal precedents in most states.

The issue of enforcement, the legal and social quandaries of traditional surrogacy, the public outcry about those arrangements following the case of Baby M, and the fact that it was challenging to find large numbers of women willing to act as traditional surrogates—any one of these could have been enough to sink surrogacy, but none of them were. Surrogacy did not cease; on the contrary, it increased. Some estimate there had been 600 surrogate births by 1988 and 6,000 by the mid-1990s (Markens 2007, 4). Two things occurred that changed the face of surrogacy, the challenge of enforcing contracts, and the dilemmas of traditional arrangements: IVF and the resulting burgeoning gestational surrogacy market.

IVF

IVF, which allows a much greater degree of control over the reproductive process, revolutionized infertility treatment. In IVF, eggs and sperm are joined in vitro—that is, in the laboratory, outside the human body. Today, fertilization commonly occurs manually, with lab workers injecting a single sperm directly into an egg in a process called intracytoplasmic sperm injection (ICSI) (Almeling 2011; Centers for Disease Control and Prevention 2011).[10] The embryos created in the laboratory are grown there, usually for three or five days, which allows REs to analyze and grade embryo quality. REs use this data to determine both which and how many embryos to transfer; if only "lower quality" embryos develop (those that are not dividing and growing well), often more embryos are transferred to increase the likelihood of success. Before the embryos are inserted into the uterus, IVF clients may opt for preimplantation genetic diagnosis (PGD) to screen for hereditary disorders. If extra embryos are created in the IVF process, they may be discarded, donated to others, or—as often occurs—frozen to be used in later rounds of IVF.

Since 1992 all US clinics that perform ART procedures have been required by Congress to provide annual data, including success rates, to the Centers for Disease Control and Prevention (2013b). Data from 2013, the most recent data available, report that 190,733 ART cycles (more than 99 percent of these are IVF procedures) were performed at 467 clinics in the United States, resulting in 54,323 births and 67,996 infants (some of the births were multiples). In other words, "approximately 1.5% of all infants born in the United States are conceived using ART" (Centers for Disease Control and Prevention 2015).

Success rates for IVF have dramatically increased since the birth of the first test-tube baby, Louise Brown, in the United Kingdom in 1978; recent estimates hover around 30 percent (Cahn 2009). Success rates, as represented by live births, vary depending on the medical conditions necessitating IVF, whether the embryos used are fresh or were frozen, and what clinic was utilized. Success rates vary most dramatically, however, based on the age of the eggs used. Egg quality decreases precipitously with age. Current live birth success rates for fresh embryo transfers using eggs from women over the age of forty-two, for example, are only 3.9 percent, while those using eggs from women under the age of thirty-five are 40.7 percent (Society for Assisted Reproductive Technology 2014).

Although the medicalization of reproduction has a long history, assisted reproduction with its various procedures and acronyms—IVF, ICSI, PGD—ushers in a new era, allowing a greater degree of control over the process and increased success, and space for multiple parties' participation in the creation of children. In 1985, four years after the first IVF birth in the United States, the first gestational surrogacy birth occurred (Andrews 1989, 5; Meinke 1988). In gestational surrogacy, the intended mother's (or the donor's) ovaries are stimulated through drug manipulation and her eggs are retrieved. The eggs are then inseminated, commonly through ICSI, in the lab with the intended father's (or donor's) sperm. For gestational surrogacy to work, the surrogate's body needs to be tricked into preparing itself for pregnancy—specifically, the uterine lining needs to be thickened, and certain hormones need to be in balance to sustain a pregnancy. The surrogate takes a sequence of fertility drugs to prepare her body for embryo transfer. At transfer, the embryos (sometimes just one) are inserted directly into the surrogate's uterus via a catheter. She is usually asked to rest following transfer—depending on the RE's preference, for a couple of hours or a couple of days. Two weeks later, the surrogate goes to the RE's office for an official pregnancy test, which measures levels of human chorionic gonadotropin (hCG) present in the blood or urine.[11] All but one of the women in my study informed me that they did not wait for the office visit, however, and took (many) home pregnancy tests during what surrogates commonly referred to as "the two-week wait."[12] If the embryos "stick" and the surrogate is pregnant, she will continue using the fertility drugs until she is released to a regular OB/GYN, usually between eight and twelve weeks' gestation.

IVF was a game changer for surrogacy. With IVF, genetic motherhood could be separated from gestation and birth. This not only allowed IPs to be the genetic parents of their children but also removed surrogates' eggs from the equation. Because of this, both surrogates and IPs have been drawn to this version of surrogacy in much greater numbers than to traditional surrogacy. Though there are still IPs who use traditional surrogacy (often because artificial insemination is cheaper than IVF) and there are women willing to act as traditional surrogates (especially because artificial insemination has a much simpler medical protocol than IVF), since IVF procedures were perfected and success rates dramatically increased, the majority of surrogacy arrangements have used IVF, not artificial insemination.

IVF has also expanded the client base of surrogacy. Whereas previously women who could not carry their own children (but produced eggs) and who did not want to use traditional surrogates might turn to adoption, foster care, or involuntary childlessness, they now have the option of hiring a woman to gestate their genetic children. Though we have no official numbers, estimates place current annual surrogacy births in the United States in the range of 1,500 (Kleinpeter 2002; Markens 2007; Teman 2010).

THE ROUTE TO PARENTHOOD

Most IPs today come to surrogacy through a route similar to the one followed by Patricia Emerson, who was profiled at the beginning of this chapter: they initially hope to carry and birth a genetically related child, but experience difficulty doing so. Some, like Patricia, have medical conditions that have compromised their uteruses. Others have been diagnosed with conditions such as lupus or severe diabetes, which are counterindicative to pregnancy. Some IPs—women born without uteruses and men who are single or gay—do not have access to the correct "parts." Unlike Patricia Emerson, however, who due to her fibroid medical condition and subsequent surgeries never attempted to get pregnant herself, many IPs have spent considerable time and economic resources attempting pregnancy.

Surrogacy is not the first preferred route to parenthood, except perhaps for gay men and women who knew prior to their childbearing years that they would be unable to achieve pregnancy. Surrogacy is not even the first option when choosing among the range of infertility treatments—it is often the last. Gestational surrogacy today is frequently found at the end of a long and expensive line of various infertility treatments that usually begin with the prescription of the drug clomiphene citrate (marketed as Clomid or Serophene) to stimulate ovulation, then move on to other drugs or surgeries (depending on the causes of infertility), intrauterine insemination (in which sperm are placed directly in the uterus), IVF, and surrogacy using IVF. Depending on the age, quality, and availability of the IPs' gametes, donated eggs and sperm are often used at various points along this trajectory.[13]

Once infertility treatment has begun—once the "reproductive team" has been assembled and IPs have been given hope that a baby, perhaps their genetic baby, awaits them at the end of the process—it is challenging to remove oneself from treatment because of the feeling that it might just be that the next drug, the next surgery, or the next treatment option will work (Cahn 2009; Mundy 2007; Spar 2006). So patients move from one treatment to the next, hopeful that their baby awaits them around the next corner. This is how many IPs find themselves at surrogacy. This was the case for Robin Clark who, after years of unsuccessful unmedicated attempts to conceive, spent five years in infertility treatments before becoming pregnant via IVF at the age of forty-five. Following the birth of her daughter, she developed an autoimmune condition. This led her and her husband, Gerald, to consider adoption as a way to bring another child into their family. Gerald, however, "got tremendous cold feet about adopting" after discussing this option with a friend of his, a friend who strongly argued for genetic parenthood. It was another of Gerald's friends who turned them onto surrogacy:

> [She] had looked all into surrogacy and explored that issue because she had two children from a previous marriage. She had just married a younger man who had never had any children whatsoever and he wanted a child of his "own blood"—kind of a crazy thing. And so she didn't want to get pregnant again because she was older and she had had difficult pregnancies, touch and go. I think she had lost a baby and, you know, no way she was going to do that! So they looked into surrogacy for his sake. And they gave us the [agency's] card. And they said, "We researched everything, this is the best place."

Though Robin felt surrogacy was an "extreme measure," especially because "there are so many children in the world [who] need a home," her husband's desire to share his genes with his offspring (a desire she saw as "kind of a crazy thing" in her husband's friends) pushed the couple toward surrogacy.

It is this ability—to conceive children who are genetically related to both intended mothers and intended fathers—that makes gestational surrogacy highly desirable for couples pursing infertility treatment. Of course, not all IPs use their own eggs and sperm in gestational surrogacy; some use the gametes of known donors or those obtained via sperm banks or egg donation agencies. But like Patricia and Robin, many IPs do intend—at least initially—to use the gametes of at least one partner when they first arrive at surrogacy as a route to parenthood.

THE CONTEMPORARY SURROGACY MARKET

The surrogacy market today in the United States includes REs who provide medical treatment, attorneys who draft and file legal papers, and for-profit agencies that recruit women to work as surrogates, match IPs and surrogates, and manage surrogacy arrangements.

Surrogacy is a small part of the infertility medical services in this country provided by a small subset of REs (not all REs include surrogacy in their practices). This is evident when looking at the few data that are available on surrogacy. For example, according to a report from the CDC (which collects annual data on reproductive medicine), less than 1 percent of all IVF cycles performed by reporting clinics in 2011 included a surrogate (Centers for Disease Control and Prevention 2011). Furthermore, the majority of the 229 clinics (out of 451) that did treat a surrogate in 2011 had very few surrogacy cases; the proportion of IVF cycles that involved a surrogate at most of these clinics was less than 2 percent. Only three clinics in the United States had double-digit surrogacy percentages (Centers for Disease Control and Prevention 2013a). For those REs who do care for surrogates, surrogacy is usually a small part of their overall practice. Infertility services for people who want to carry their own pregnancy themselves instead of employing a surrogate constitute REs' bread and butter.

Infertility clinics tend to cluster together geographically. The largest clusters appear in only seven states, with California having by far the most (sixty-four) clinics that provided infertility services in 2011. The other states include Texas (thirty-nine clinics), New York (thirty-eight), Florida (twenty-eight), and Illinois (twenty-six). Some states (Arkansas, Idaho, Montana, New Mexico, North Dakota, Rhode Island, South Dakota, and Vermont) only have one clinic; Maine has none (Centers for Disease Control and Prevention 2013a). Six states (California, Illinois, Massachusetts, New Jersey, New York, and Texas) account for almost half of all ART procedures (48 percent) and live births from ART (46 percent) in the United States (Sunderam et al. 2014). This helps explain the clustering of surrogacy medical services as well. For example, surromomsonline.com, a popular surrogacy website, lists twenty-eight infertility clinics offering surrogacy services (quite a few with multiple locations) in California, while no clinic is listed for Michigan, a state that bans commercial surrogacy. In these variations across the country, the impact of infertility services in general and differences in states' friendliness to surrogacy are visible.

Some REs also develop reputations as surrogacy-friendly and receive referrals from agencies and attorneys. IP clients and surrogates are also important purveyors of such referrals. This was the case with Randall Blackborne, an RE with whom I spoke. Randall and his clinic have become a popular destination for IPs and surrogates seeking IVF services. When I asked him how he came to work in surrogacy, he told me:

> It just kind of started. Someone came here and they had failed [to conceive] at several other places and they saw that we had very high success rates for IVF so they thought, "Oh why don't we give it a go there?" And it worked for the gestational carrier. And then there have been several news stories that have been done on TV. So I think people see it that way. I think that there's this whole group of Internet chat rooms or something that goes on amongst these groups and they talk amongst themselves and say, "Oh yeah, Dr. Blackborne has done a lot of these things. Why don't you go see him?" So we have people coming from all over the country. I'm assuming it's the Internet that's getting that information out because I'm not going out there saying, "Hey! Come on in!" It's just kind of happening.

As Randall suggests, much of the surrogacy recruitment and advertising takes place on the Internet. Not only do agencies, attorneys, and REs (even Randall) have websites and advertise their services on line, but there are also websites (such as surromomsonline.com and allaboutsurrogacy.com) that interested parties can search for information and use to meet each other.

Some surrogates and IPs who find each other online go on to manage surrogacy journeys themselves, without the use of a surrogacy agency. An independent arrangement (known in the surrogacy community as an "indy") sometimes occurs between known parties: for example, an aunt could carry a baby for her niece, often for no monetary compensation. Other indy arrangements are between parties who meet each other via friends or through the surrogacy community, especially via Internet websites where IPs and surrogates can post classified ads. There is no accurate way to know how many indy or agency arrangements occur in the United States. However, anecdotal evidence from surrogacy professionals and surrogates suggests that the market is dominated by for-profit agencies.

There is considerable variation among surrogacy agencies in terms of the types of surrogacy arrangements they offer (traditional and gestational), how much they charge, and the services they provide. These variations are due to the lack of federal oversight and the impact of different state legislation or case law, levels of experience, ethics and standards, and amounts of resources. Surrogacy agencies are not required by the federal government to follow specific practices. There are only a handful of agencies that have decades of experiences. These agencies have large lists of clients and maybe a dozen full-time employees and a handful of part-time screeners or coordinators. There are also many newer smaller agencies: over 120 agencies, for example, advertise on surromomsonline. com. Many of these smaller agencies are not much more than a website and a home office run by one or two people who outsource any services (especially legal services or psychological testing) they require. The larger agencies have set the tone and industry standards for the practice of surrogacy. Smaller agencies often piggyback on the success of the larger ones by duplicating their rhetoric, rules, even materials (such as websites—which sometimes gets them into legal trouble).

Many agencies, both large and small, are run by former—occasionally current—surrogates or IPs. The larger ones sometimes have an egg donation program, affiliated legal staff members, psychologists or counselors who evaluate surrogates and run support groups, coordinators for both IPs and surrogates, and screeners who interview applicants. Some surrogacy agencies also handle adoptions, foster care arrangements, or egg donation. Some surrogacy programs are embedded in law practices or RE clinics; many others are stand-alone entities.

The three main players on the professional side of surrogacy—agencies, attorneys, and REs—establish working relationships with each other. Agencies often have particular legal or RE practices with whom they like to work and which they recommend to their IP clients—and vice versa. There are certain tasks associated with each player, though sometimes an agency will have attorneys on staff and also handle the legal aspects, or an RE's office will perform the duties handled by agencies, such as matching IPs and surrogates and facilitating psychological testing. For example, one attorney, James Ianson, explained that though he handles the legal paperwork for surrogacy agencies, especially those in other states, he also matches IP clients with surrogates. Thus, the role he plays in surrogacy arrangements can vary considerably: for some IP-surrogate partners he functions as the matchmaker, broker, agency director, and attorney, while for others his role is limited to that of the attorney who reviews and files the surrogacy legal documents.

Agencies, attorneys, and REs often have contacts with each other as a surrogacy journey progresses. Raquel Marklin, who manages James's surrogacy program, explained how that program and REs work simultaneously with an IP couple, relying on each other to keep the surrogacy on "the up and up." Before REs "move forward with an embryo transfer or even retrieval," Raquel told me, "they have to have a clearance from us. A lot of them want to make sure that the contract has been signed and everything is fine on this end before they move forward on that end."

The contract Raquel was referring to is one of the two important legal documents filed in gestational surrogacy arrangements. Contracts are signed by both IPs and surrogates and give the specifics of their arrangements. Contracts have evolved from the one-page agreements used in traditional surrogacies in the early 1980s to today's thirty-page documents that are full of legal jargon delineating all aspects of the arrangement: not only the primary objective of specifying the child's parentage, but also such issues as compensation, financial responsibility, and the number of embryos to be transferred. Sometimes contracts include minutiae such as the number of cups of coffee the surrogate can drink per day or restrictions on the use of certain foods or cleaning products. Contracts also usually include important decisions about "what if" scenarios, such as: What if the surrogate ends up carrying more fetuses than anticipated (for example, two embryos are transferred and they both split, creating quadruplets), and the RE believes the situation to make a healthy baby outcome unlikely—will two of those fetuses be selectively reduced? What if prenatal tests indicate there is a high possibility of Down syndrome—will the fetus be aborted? What if the surrogate goes into premature labor and needs bed rest—will the IPs pay for lost wages and child care for her children? Attorneys not only ensure that contracts are properly signed and filed but also counsel IPs and surrogates about these and other negotiating points and stipulations.

The negotiation process and the contract phase can be extended or abbreviated. This may depend on whether or not the IPs and surrogate are using the same attorney or if they have separate legal counsel. Sometimes agencies with affiliated legal staff members will recommend that both parties use their attorneys. Some agencies require IPs and surrogates not to use the same attorneys.[14] Sometimes surrogates forgo legal counsel or use the same attorney as their IPs to save the IPs money (IPs usually pay for all legal services associated with the surrogacy).

The second important document handled by attorneys in surrogacy arrangements is the prebirth order—the legal document that is filed before the birth of the child to allow the IPs' names to be put on the birth certificate at the hospital, rather than the surrogate's name (and her husband's, if she is married). Not all jurisdictions allow prebirth orders, but for those that do, the proper filing of this document is important for both IPs and surrogates as it makes the surrogate's postbirth relinquishment of maternal rights and adoption by a second parent unnecessary. For those couples who do not have a prebirth order, attorneys will handle the paperwork associated with the transfer of parental rights from the surrogate to the IPs after the birth.

Attorneys also sometimes set up and manage surrogacy escrow accounts through which funds are distributed to surrogates and sometimes to surrogacy agencies. These accounts are often required by agencies so that they and the surrogates are ensured that funds are available and in trust to pay for associated procedures and to compensate the surrogate. Many surrogacy programs require IPs to deposit all of the necessary funds into an escrow account at the beginning of the surrogacy journey. Attorneys then manage these accounts, distributing the funds as deemed appropriate according to the contract.

Some surrogacy attorneys have reproductive law practices, focusing on surrogacy and egg or embryo donation. Others are family law attorneys who also handle traditional adoptions and divorce. For still others, surrogacy may be a small part of their practice, with the main part in another area of law. Some attorneys, like James Ianson, own and run surrogacy programs; others are affiliated with a surrogacy agency; still others' law firms are separate from any agency.

For this book, I spoke with surrogacy professionals like James Ianson and Randall Blackborne: agency directors, counselors, psychologists, surrogacy coordinators, screeners, attorneys, and medical practitioners who work for or with large, established agencies and much smaller and newer ones. These interviews highlighted for me the variations that exist among surrogacy professionals: not every attorney follows the same procedures, not every agency handles surrogates in the same way, and not every RE has the same experience dealing with surrogacy or prescribes the same medical protocol. While REs have organizations that provide recommendations for the medical practices related to surrogacy, neither REs nor attorneys are bound by particular surrogacy regulations. Attorneys and REs, however, do have professional rules and codes of conduct they must follow regarding the practice of law and medicine, respectively, to be licensed. They have passed board exams required by their professions, and they face having their licenses revoked should they engage in behavior that is deemed professionally unethical. Surrogacy agencies and their owners exist in a different realm: one that has no licensing, accreditation, or advanced degree requirements. Anyone can hang out a shingle and declare herself or himself the director of a surrogacy agency. There are no regulatory forces in place to prevent inexperienced or unscrupulous people from brokering surrogacy arrangements.

This unregulated wild West aspect of surrogacy agency brokers is evident in several recent high-profile cases. In 2011, for example, it was discovered that Hilary Neiman, a Maryland attorney who ran a surrogacy agency, operated what the Federal Bureau of Investigation (FBI) called a "surrogacy scam" with Theresa Erickson, a well-known California surrogacy attorney, and Carla Chambers, an alleged former nurse from New Zealand who acted as the surrogate coordinator (Federal Bureau of Investigation 2011). These three found women via surrogacy websites and classified ads and flew them to Ukraine to become impregnated with already created donor embryos. Once the pregnancies had been established, the three would then match the pregnant women with IPs (Zarembo 2011). According to the FBI, the IPs "were told the unborn babies were the result of legitimate surrogacy arrangements, but the original IPs had backed out. They were offered the opportunity to 'assume' the nonexistent surrogacy agreement" for between $100,000 and $150,000 (Federal Bureau of Investigation 2011). Neiman and Erickson would then create fraudulent paperwork, including prebirth orders, stating that the surrogacy arrangement had existed before the pregnancy, which Neiman would file in California. The impregnated women reportedly thought they were engaging in legitimate surrogacy. Neither the surrogates nor the IPs, according to the FBI, were aware that they were engaged in illegal baby selling. All three coconspirators were sentenced to serve prison time, home confinement, and/or pay fines (Federal Bureau of Investigation 2012).

In another recent high-profile case, the owner of a Modesto, California, agency called SurroGenesis scammed her clients and surrogates out of funds via their escrow accounts. According to the FBI, Tonya Collins "steered Surrogenesis [sic] clients to Michael Charles Independent Financial but concealed her ownership and operation of the escrow company, including creating fictitious employee identities to make it appear that Michael Charles was an independent company with its own staff." Instead of using clients' funds to pay for necessary surrogacy expenses, Collins spent over $2 million for "unauthorized personal purchases: automobiles, homes, jewelry, clothing, and vacations for herself and others, without the clients' knowledge or consent" (Federal Bureau of Investigation 2013a). Because all of their surrogacy-designated funds had disappeared, some SurroGenesis IP clients who were in the middle of their surrogacy pregnancies were unable to pay their surrogates; others at earlier stages were unable to continue their quest for parenthood (Saul 2009). In May 2013, Collins was found guilty of wire fraud and sentenced to five years and three months in prison. She was also ordered to pay restitution to each victim (Federal Bureau of Investigation 2013b).

These types of scandals, involving unscrupulous exploitation and blatant greed, highlight the vulnerabilities in surrogacy practice that, coupled with the large amounts of money involved and the lack of regulation and licensing, make it tempting to criminals. Due to such scandals, especially following the case of Baby M, it has become common in the surrogacy market for professionals to follow, or purport to follow, certain informal rules. These rules are designed to protect surrogacy and surrogacy players from scandals, litigation, and public scrutiny.

The first important rule involves clients' funds. Many agencies insist that independent escrow companies manage clients' funds. This is supposed to provide assurance to IPs that their funds are being managed properly and to both surrogates and agencies that there will be funds available to disburse when they are needed. Another rule involves contracts. Though there are some (mostly independent instead of agency-managed) surrogacies that take place purely after an oral agreement, most agencies and RE clinics—regardless of the legal status of surrogacy in their state, which may make contracts unenforceable—insist that contracts be finalized before any medical procedures take place.

These established rules attempt to provide a structure for a practice that largely exists in a gray legal area. As various surrogacy scandals demonstrate, however, the rules are not always followed, and there is actually nothing in place to ensure that they are obeyed. True regulation of agency structure and practice (such as how funds are managed and designating who is able to own and manage a surrogacy agency) would require institutionalized regulation and sanctions overseen by either a universally recognized professional organization of surrogacy agencies (which does not exist) or the federal government (which is not making any movement toward surrogacy regulation).

Regulation would severely curtail the practice of surrogacy and challenge the free-market mentality that currently exists. Many surrogacy professionals understand, however, that they must manage the image of surrogacy, protect themselves from litigation, and limit the number of scandals if their own businesses and the surrogacy market as a whole are going to prosper. Therefore, there are additional rules in the surrogacy market—although most of them focus not on agency structure or limiting the market, but on who is allowed to participate in surrogacy as an IP or a surrogate.

RULES FOR INTENDED PARENTS

Intended parents are the clients of surrogacy agencies. Therefore, few rules apply to their participation in surrogacy. They must be able to pay for services, and agencies will often verify that they have adequate financial resources to do so. Surrogacy fees, like the practice of surrogacy itself, are unregulated. Depending on what types of treatment and services are necessary, a surrogacy journey can cost upward of $150,000, if medical costs are included and especially if the IPs are not successful the first time (which is not unusual). However, the range of costs associated with surrogacy, each dependent on different service providers, results in a wide variation in the bottom line.

Medical fees account for a large part of the expense of surrogacy: fees for REs (for IVF) and for OB/GYNs and hospitals (for prenatal care, birth, and postnatal care). In the United States, a single IVF cycle alone averages $12,400 (American Society for Reproductive Medicine n.d.). It is not unusual for IPs to need more than one cycle to achieve a live birth. Medical fees can vary widely. For example, a journey involving a surrogate who gets pregnant following the first transfer of an embryo that was created using her IPs' gametes and who has an unproblematic pregnancy and an uncomplicated vaginal birth of a healthy singleton will have much lower fees associated with conception, pregnancy, and birth than a journey involving a surrogate who needs four embryo transfers, trying first with her IPs' gametes but then moving onto donor eggs and then donor eggs and sperm (all of which must be paid for); who becomes pregnant with twins (for which there is often an added fee of $5,000–$8,000 that goes to the surrogate); who develops gestational diabetes and needs to spend three months on bed rest (which often involves an added fee for the surrogate as well as fees for her house and child care and lost wages reimbursement if she has outside employment); and who has an emergency cesarean section at thirty weeks' gestation, with the babies spending two months in the neonatal intensive care unit. Journeys similar to both of these scenarios occur in surrogacy. At the beginning of a surrogacy journey, IPs, REs, and agencies often do not know how complicated or long the process to a live birth will be for a particular couple. Therefore, agencies attempt to ensure that IPs have adequate financial resources to provide for the contingencies common in IVF surrogacy.

Portions of the medical care involved in surrogacy, such as prenatal care and birth, are sometimes covered by a surrogate's medical insurance if her policy does not have a surrogacy exclusion (which disallows maternal coverage to women gestating children for surrogacy).[15] Insurance coverage for assisted reproduction, however, is unusual in the United States—even for basic IVF, let alone the use of a surrogate—and most IPs must pay for these services themselves (American Society for Reproductive Medicine 2010; Becker 2000).

IPs are also responsible for attorney fees associated with their surrogacy. These fees vary depending on the surrogate's state of residence, whether or not any complications are involved in the particular situation, the level of negotiation needed during the contract phase, and whether or not the IPs use an agency's in-house attorney. I have seen attorney fees for surrogacy advertised for as little as $2,000 and for as much as $12,500.

IPs who use an agency must also pay for its services. Agency-associated fees for surrogacy can be divided into several parts. First is the agency's fee, which can range from $10,000 to $20,000. Then there is surrogate compensation, which is often a negotiated figure and can therefore vary widely. Agency employees and surrogates informed me that surrogate fees average from $15,000 to $25,000 for first-time surrogates and from $20,000 to $35,000 for experienced surrogates. Surrogate fees also vary depending on the state where the surrogate lives (California surrogates often receive higher fees, reportedly due to their higher cost of living) and whether or not the surrogate has her own medical insurance that will cover prenatal care and birth. Surrogates whose insurance does cover a surrogacy pregnancy usually receive higher fees; otherwise, IPs need to buy an insurance rider, find a policy for the surrogate, or pay for those medical expenses out of pocket.

Surrogates are not expected to pay for any fees associated with the surrogacy; any expenses incurred are the responsibility of the IPs. Therefore, in addition to compensation, surrogates are often reimbursed for travel expenses, child care, and housekeeping services; given allowances for maternity clothing; and remunerated for support-group attendance, which is sometimes mandatory. Most medical procedures also have surrogate fees attached. For example, if the surrogate undergoes a cesarean section, she may receive $4,000; if she has amniocentesis, $400; and if she suffers a miscarriage, $600. These fees are negotiated, usually ironed out during the contract phase or set by the individual agencies, and therefore vary.

Finally, IPs are responsible for the fees associated with the psychological testing and counseling for them and their surrogate that many agencies and REs require for participation in their programs. These fees—from $1,000 to $4,000—are sometimes included in the overall agency fee but other times are separate.

Due to variation in both individual IPs' journeys and the fee structures of agencies, attorneys, and REs, it is challenging to place a typical price tag on surrogacy. The nonmedical portion of surrogacy (covering agency, surrogate, psychological, and legal fees) may range between $60,000 and $80,000, and the medical portion (including testing) may be an additional $20,000–$30,000 per IVF cycle—with many IPs needing more than one cycle to achieve pregnancy. To ensure that their clients can pay for these services, surrogacy agencies will run credit checks and sometimes refer IPs to loan specialists, encourage home mortgage refinancing and the use of credit, and have links to banks on their websites.

As it is currently practiced in the United States, commercial surrogacy is therefore largely available as a route to parenthood only to people with considerable means or with access to enough credit (or sympathetic relatives) to cover the costs. The cost of surrogacy, which considerably reduces the infertile population able to afford these services, is similar to the costs of advanced reproductive technologies as a whole. The result is that treatment for infertility in the United States is overwhelmingly a middle- and upper-class phenomenon (Becker 2000; Bell 2014; Rapp 1997).

In addition to concerns regarding potential IP clients' ability to pay for services, many agencies will also screen IPs for anticipated problematic behavior and attitudes, as agencies want surrogacy arrangements to function smoothly. Sometimes the screening process is not much more than making a phone call or requiring IPs to complete an online survey; other times it involves multiple consultations with various agency employees, a criminal background check, and psychological screening. If the screening indicates problematic behavior—for example, if IPs appear to be overly controlling or unrealistically demanding, or if it seems as though they will need an overabundance of hand-holding or will otherwise consume more than their share of an agency's time and resources, then agencies will sometimes deny them entry into their programs. Sometimes agency directors "listen to their gut" and encourage IPs to look elsewhere for services. Several agency directors and owners informed me that they have refused to work with IPs who displayed "extreme prejudice" or who wanted to engage in behavior they thought was unethical. Janice Holberg, for example, the director of a large established agency, told me of a couple who informed her during the initial IP screening that they would terminate the pregnancy if their gestating fetus turned out to be female. When the intended father informed her of the reason (he "needed an heir"), she said to him, "You know what? I just don't think that we're the right agency for you." Janice told me, "I just didn't want to accept somebody with that kind of attitude." Other agencies reject potential clients based on their marital status or sexual orientation. This depends heavily on agency location, state legislation or case law, agency viability, and—as with the intended father Janice refused to serve—case-by-case judgments by agency directors.

Beyond screening IPs for the ability to pay for services and temperament, the most consistent rule governing IPs' participation in surrogacy is that many surrogacy professionals (agencies and REs) will work only with IPs who face challenges achieving pregnancy and birthing a live child themselves. Surrogacy is framed as a solution to infertility, not as an alternative route to gestational parenthood, which is the current framing used in adoption (Jacobson 2008). Surrogacy is specifically framed as second best—an option that is not preferred but that allows IPs to achieve what they do prefer: genetic parenthood and the experience (at least by proxy) of pregnancy. In fact, the overriding narrative of the marketing campaign to attract IPs is that surrogacy allows one to experience one's own pregnancy via the body of a surrogate. It is the IPs' baby and the IPs' pregnancy, not the surrogate's, participants in my study told me. In agency materials used to attract prospective clients, there is an emphasis on the biological connections with the child available through gestational surrogacy that parents cannot have in other routes, especially adoption.

Though adoption is seldom mentioned in surrogacy materials or in discussions I have had with surrogacy professionals, the surrogacy market tries to reach clients who are on their way out of the RE's office, off the gestational pregnancy track, and who may be heading toward adoption or involuntary childlessness. Recall Robin Clark and her husband, Gerald: after finally birthing their daughter via IVF and five years on the "infertility train," Robin and Gerald were turning toward adoption to expand their family. They were pulled back to the RE's office, however, by the lure of gestational parenthood for Gerald (at that point Robin's eggs were deemed too old to be used). Like Robin, many intended mothers have exhausted the range of infertility treatments leading to pregnancy via their own bodies by the time the idea of surrogacy arises. Recall also when Patricia Emerson's RE informed her that she had no hope of carrying a pregnancy herself. We could imagine Patricia then turning toward adoption. Patricia noted that she was unfamiliar with surrogacy and the mechanics of how to find a surrogate for herself. Her RE, however, quickly stepped in and suggested surrogacy as the solution. This is the path that brings many IPs to surrogacy. A common narrative that people shared with me is that after failed attempts at a fertility clinic, a physician or the client will initiate a discussion about surrogacy, during which the physician will give the client contact information for an agency or listing of agencies with whom the physician has worked—or, if an RE matches IPs and surrogates, he or she may offer that service. This allows the RE to retain clients and continue their treatment—though through the addition of a third party. It is often through their RE that IPs gain knowledge about surrogacy and particular agencies.

The initial treatment relationship between IPs and REs is also the route through which agencies gain confirmation that IPs are truly infertile. Though agencies state that they will work only with IP clients who cannot birth children themselves, agencies often do not review IPs' medical records. Deidre Richards, a former surrogate and the owner of a small surrogacy agency, let me know that this was the case with her company. Instead, she told me, "I figured if a fertility clinic is referring somebody to me, they've worked with them a while and done some testing and know that they're pretty legit."

The decision to work with only "legit" clients began early on in contracted surrogacy arrangements; we can see the need for this rule arising after the case of Baby M. Embedded in media critiques of that case were implications that Elizabeth Stern, the intended mother, did not legitimately need surrogacy: her multiple sclerosis was "mild," and she simply "did not want to risk complications" ("Who's Who in the Fight for Baby M" 1987). Indeed, we could imagine similar framings of a contemporary client seeking surrogate services because she wants to avoid the pains of pregnancy; and in this age of what Arlie Hochschild calls the "commodity frontier," in which the market develops "commercial substitutes for family activities" (2003, 37), we could imagine a surrogacy market that would be amenable to those types of arrangements. In fact, there has been recent discussion in the media of agencies changing course and working with IPs who have social, not medical, challenges to pregnancy. In April 2014, the California agency Conceptual Options was profiled on ABC News, with its director, the psychologist Saira Jhutty, quoted as stating that she has IP clients who choose surrogacy because they are "afraid of being pregnant," "work in an industry where image is very important," or "don't want to have to go through the changes that happen to a woman's body when they get pregnant" (ABC News 2014). Another agency director, Karen Synesiou of the Center for Surrogate Parenting, was quoted in a recent front-page story in the *New York Times* (Lewin 2014) as stating that although her agency "usually only take[s] clients who have a medical need," it has recently begun accepting "government officials" from China as IP clients who "would be in trouble if they break the one-child rule." Synesiou called this "political surrogacy." While these cases have garnered media interest, critics of commercial surrogacy often imply that such scenarios, with the privileged class renting the wombs of the underclass to avoid the social and physical discomfort of pregnancy and still achieve genetic parenthood, constitutes the majority of the surrogacy market.

Most surrogacy brokers are familiar with this criticism and aim to disempower it through working only with clients who have medical needs. This is in line with the recommendations of the American Society for Reproductive Medicine, which state: "Gestational carriers may be used when a true medical condition precludes the intended parent from carrying a pregnancy or would pose a significant risk of death or harm to the woman or the fetus" (2012a, 1301).

The focus on needs-based clients places IPs—especially intended mothers—as worthy of what those in the world of surrogacy like to call the "gift of surrogacy." Intended mothers are often framed in the surrogacy community as having made sacrifices in their attempts at motherhood. This aligns nicely with traditional notions of motherhood in which "good mothers" sacrifice themselves (their bodies, their time, and their own needs) on behalf of their children (Damaske 2011; Hays 1996; Malacrida and Boulton 2012). The use of a surrogate cannot be based on a desire to rent a uterus for convenience's sake; instead, it must be because the intended mother is physically incapable of gestating a child herself.

Clients with medical needs challenge the framing of surrogacy as crass commercialization of the uterus with their stories of repeated miscarriages, fetal deaths, and stillbirths that pull on the heartstrings and position surrogacy as a solution to seemingly unending heartache. Most agencies abide by this rule of serving only needs-based clients to deflect detractors and toe the line of industry standards. Besides being able to pay for services, being needs-based is the main rule IPs must follow for inclusion in surrogacy. However, the main regulatory focus of surrogacy is not the IPs, it is the surrogates.

Rules for Surrogates

While there are few rules governing IP participation, there are many for potential surrogates. These rules vary from agency to agency, but several are fairly standard in the US market. The first is that women wanting to become surrogates must have birthed and mothered a child. This rule was explained to me as achieving two specific objectives. The first is to demonstrate to agencies and REs that a potential surrogate has what they call a "proven uterus"—that she is a known quantity in terms of her ability to achieve and sustain a pregnancy. Surrogacy is not cheap; IPs are spending considerable sums attempting to achieve a live birth. The medical protocol is quite complex, and one gets fairly far into the process before the official pregnancy test occurs. REs and agencies (and many IPs themselves) therefore prefer to work with surrogates who are known to be able to birth live infants.

Surrogacy professionals prefer to work with women who have had unproblematic pregnancies, but the specific details about what constitutes such a pregnancy vary from agency to agency and from RE to RE. For example, some will work only with women who have birthed vaginally, while others accept women who have had multiple cesarean sections; some refuse to work with women who have had miscarriages, gestational diabetes, or who have a higher body mass index (BMI), while others allow such women into their programs. However, requiring a surrogate to have demonstrated her ability to achieve and maintain a pregnancy and to birth a live child is a rule followed by many agencies and RE clinics in the United States.

The second objective to accepting as surrogates only women who have birthed and mothered a child is to minimize the possibility that a surrogate might want to keep the surro-baby. Here the ghost of Baby M can be seen to continue to haunt surrogacy, as agencies attempt to avoid any similar cases. The hope is that because surrogates have previously given birth, they will understand what is involved in motherhood and enter into surrogate arrangements with their eyes open. Cheryl Woodley, the director of a large agency, explained why her agency works only with women who have birthed and mothered a child:

> Isn't it better that a surrogate mom has done this once and understands that her bonding is not with the concept of a child but with her child, with her genetics? And the [surrogate] child she gives birth to, she knows as she goes through the pregnancy it's a different kind of a bonding and, "Yeah, I could give this child to the couple. I could give them back their baby." You don't know if you could do that if you've never had a child. And why would we [force her to give the child to the IPs]? Because we're contractually obligated to make her do that. I don't want to hurt her, I don't want to hurt the couple, but my goodness, she had no idea she would feel this way. So that's the one thing. I think every surrogate mom should have given birth.

Having experienced birth and parenthood should give surrogates, Cheryl argued, enough of an understanding of motherhood to realize that the children they gestate in surrogacy are not their children, not their "genetics." She seems to believe that true maternal bonding, occurring during pregnancy and birth, is possible only with genetic motherhood. This framing posits that realizing surrogate children are not surrogates' children is what allows surrogates to "return" the children to their "true parents," the IPs.

This reification of biological bonds is a dramatic turn from traditional surrogacy, in which the genetics of the children were downplayed (because the surrogates were the genetic mothers) and the intent of the parents was emphasized. Intent is still important in gestational surrogacy—especially when egg or sperm donors are used—but as Cheryl's comments make clear, these new IVF arrangements allow for a reiteration of parenthood via genetic bonds that is not possible in other alternative routes to motherhood such as adoption, egg donation, or traditional surrogacy. Here we can see that gestational surrogacy, which appears on the surface to transgress traditional ideologies of the family, actually reinforces notions of the strength of biological kinship ties. The children created via gestational surrogacy are conceptualized by the surrogacy market and surrogacy players as truly the IPs' progeny because they are created from the IPs' gametes. The surrogate's maternity status toward the surrogate child needs to be obliterated for commercial surrogacy to operate and flourish. Otherwise, surrogacy is an arrangement in which women are being paid to relinquish their maternal rights and sell their babies, which is not only illegal but culturally unpalatable. Surrogates must therefore be mothers to their own children, surrogacy professionals informed me, so that they truly understand that they are not mothers to the surro-babies they gestate.

Another common rule used by agencies in the selection of surrogates is to exclude women on government assistance. Several justifications for this rule were given to me. Some professionals noted that surrogate work would jeopardize families' benefits (because welfare recipients must report any income). Other agency directors avoid women in economic distress, which they viewed as stressful for the body and potentially resulting in negative impacts on pregnancy. Still others saw financial instability as a potential source of strain in the surrogate-IP relationship. Janice Holberg explained that surrogates "need to be financially independent themselves because if they're on public assistance, they're very dependent on that public assistance. What if they don't get pregnant and receive this money? And what if they don't get a transfer fee, they don't make it as far as a transfer—and they're devastated because financially they're not going to be able to make it? Well, then, the couple is going to feel obligated to help out." This rule, according to Janice, is based on concern for IPs. Agencies do not want their IP clients to feel obligated to support surrogates financially—which would be quite possible, I was told, if an agency accepted women on public assistance.

These three explanations for the rule against welfare recipients—impact on the surrogate's welfare benefits, impact on the surrogate's body, and impact on the IP-surrogate relationship—focus on the internal dynamics of ensuring successful journeys. However, when I asked Cheryl Woodley if the rule against welfare mothers was "because of the stress and instability" on the surrogate's body, she shook her head and answered:

No, I think part of it is, as a professional in the field, I know that's one thing I can be attacked on by female libbers et cetera. That you're working with poor people who are doing this for the money. It's just one less thing I've got to deal with if I don't do that. They can't attack me on that because no, I don't work with people who are on welfare. That's not who we qualify surrogate moms as. But it's more about us being attacked, quite frankly. I mean we created the rule a long time ago because we were attacked in the very early days by [people] saying, "Surrogate moms are poor, underprivileged ladies that will do anything to feed their families." And maybe those are the ones who should be surrogate moms because they need the help more than anything else. I just know I can't touch them because it's not right for our field. Maybe we wouldn't exist had we done that.

According to Cheryl, the survival of her agency, and perhaps of surrogacy practice as a whole, hinged on having a specific wholesome image of surrogates to present to the outside world: women who are above scrutiny, are financially stable, love being pregnant, and want to help infertile couples achieve parenthood. And this, by and large, is what I found.

The typical woman in my study was a married lower- or middle-class woman with several children, who had some college education but no degree, who works outside the home in a female-dominated profession, and who loves pregnancy. As I will discuss in the following chapter, all of the surrogates in my study spoke of their enjoyment of pregnancy and the joy they derived from giving IPs their much desired children. An important part of that image, according to Cheryl and other surrogacy professionals, was ensuring that surrogates do not appear desperate—that they engage in surrogacy not out of economic necessity, not because they are being exploited to use their bodies for pay, but out of an innate desire to help others.

The motivations of surrogates are complex: as I show in the next chapter, they include an interesting mix of internal and external factors. However, the marketing discourse used to draw women into the field—and to weed out undesirable applicants—emphasizes the gift-giving nature of surrogacy. Surrogacy as the ultimate gift, the rhetoric claims, is not baby selling or renting one's womb out of crass monetary greed. It is not work in the sense that one is engaging in it simply to make an income: the heart is involved. By framing surrogacy as a gift given to truly needy infertile couples by warmhearted, financially stable, loving mothers, surrogacy market players are attempting to manage the impression of surrogacy. By arguing that surrogacy is a gift, the market attempts to obscure both the work involved in and the income generated from surrogacy. Surrogacy agencies, like many businesses in the public eye that receive scrutiny, desire to avoid bad press—in this case, the bad publicity that comes from negative framings of surrogacy and from controversial, problematic, and litigious surrogacy cases.

These two rules—having birthed and mothered a child and not being on welfare—are rules consistently applied to surrogates in the market, which help to legitimize surrogacy. These rules could leave many women eligible, however, and many women, surrogate professionals tell me, would not make good surrogates. There are specific qualities beyond being a financially stable mother that agencies, especially the large, well-established ones, search for in their surrogates.

Agencies attempt to attract high-quality surrogates to their programs. The agency directors in my study—especially from the larger programs—spoke of receiving an overabundance of applications from women wanting to work as surrogates. Agency directors and employees discussed the need to weed out rather than recruit applicants. Samantha Miller, a surrogate screener, explained that in her agency "only four out of every one hundred applicants are actually accepted. And out of those four, maybe two will actually become surrogates. So the percentage of our applicants that actually become surrogates is very small."

Agencies look for women who take their medications correctly and on time, can follow the complicated medical protocol, do not complain, do not cause a fuss, and "do as they are told"—in other words, women who are compliant workers. Women with substance abuse issues (or whose husbands or intimate partners have such issues) are ruled out; but also problematic are those with higher BMIs, recent tattoos, antidepressant use, unsupportive spouses, and police records. Potential surrogates have medical examinations of their uteruses and tests of their general health to ensure that medically they are good candidates for IVF. Most programs also have age restrictions, looking for women between the ages of twenty-one and forty or forty-two (though some older surrogates in my study had successfully completed multiple journeys). The initial screening process of potential surrogates usually includes asking about these details, and credit and criminal background checks are run.

In looking for good workers, agencies attempt to find women who will take the work seriously, think of surrogacy as their job, and comply with the complicated protocol and sometimes tricky social dynamics. When I posed the question "Do surrogates think about surrogacy as work?" to Janice Holberg, the agency director, she replied: "I hope so! Because we do kind of explain it to them: 'This is your job.' In fact we had a surrogate who was a social worker too. She was going to take a second job and we said, 'Your second job is your surrogacy!' She wanted the missed wages for the second job, and we said no: 'Surrogacy is your second job, and it's not fair to ask the couple to pay missed wages for a third job.'" Like Janice, other surrogacy brokers want their surrogates to consider surrogacy their job, to invest the time and effort in it that one does in a job (even a second job). Ironically, however, they also want surrogates not to think of surrogacy as employment in the sense of it being an income-generating position. Though they use compensation as a recruitment tool—and surrogates do earn money from surrogacy, as I will discuss in later chapters—agencies do not want women who are primarily motivated by money, preferring that they see their compensation as a gift from their IPs, not a paycheck.

To try to elicit the true motivations of potential surrogates, many agencies have applicants meet with psychologists or counselors. The women take standardized psychological tests such as the Minnesota Multiphasic Personality Inventory (MMPI) and talk with counselors about their motivations. Surrogacy psychologists, counselors, and agency directors let me know that part of the objective of the psychological evaluation is to weed out women who are just in it for the money, for as many people in this study—both surrogacy professionals and surrogates—told me, money is not enough of a motivating factor to keep surrogates compliant. You cannot do surrogacy for the money, they told me; there is just too much work involved. If you are only doing it for the money, they reiterated, you might not comply with the work requirements. The heart, not only the pocketbook, must be involved.

Martha Griffin, a psychologist who screens potential surrogates for a large surrogacy program, let me know that finding surrogates with nonmonetary motivations was an important aspect of agency work. "You have to have good surrogates," Martha reported, women motivated by a "giving heart" who view surrogacy as a gift. For agencies to survive, they have to have good workers. Ironically, a good worker is one who does not make it obvious that she is working, that she is collecting a paycheck to grow this baby. Rather, good workers are compliant, kind, and giving—women who would appear to be people who just might engage in this labor without receiving compensation. Good workers put up with a lot—because they care. Martha elaborated: "You have to be doing it for more than the money or else you just can't sustain the drama, the pain, the disappointments, the social disapproval, the sacrifices you're making. So even if it's for the money—and I don't have many of those surrogates, but I have some. I've certainly met them outside of [my agency]. You take on other reasons because it's just too darned hard."

The screening process for surrogates, figuring out who has the right stuff to engage in work that is "just too darned hard" is an important aspect of the industry. The industry rules that have been developed to govern who is chosen to work as surrogates—women who have proven uteruses, who have mothered their own children, and who are psychologically sound and financially stable— attempt to mitigate any potential obstacles that might arise in the process. The selection process is meant to protect IPs (the clients) and agencies themselves from the multiple potential heartbreaks and disasters that could arise in surrogacy due to its status in legal limbo: the surrogate unable to get pregnant, the surrogate who absconds with a gestating fetus or who moves to a surrogacy-unfriendly state to have herself declared its mother, who extorts money from her IPs, or, perhaps most devastatingly, who complies with everything but then demands the baby in the end—another Mary Beth Whitehead.

By demonstrating to IP clients that they use a highly selective process to choose their surrogates, agencies attempt to signal their legitimacy. This legitimization is increasingly important as the field expands and various scandals receive publicity. Since its inception, surrogacy has existed in a legal gray area. High-profile cases, such as those of SurroGenesis and the baby-selling ring, have kept surrogacy on unsure footing. This is a problem for surrogacy professionals when they attempt to recruit IP clients and surrogate workers. Demonstrating that they have strict standards for surrogate selection is one way an agency can separate itself from unsavory agencies and establish the legitimacy of its practice.

Conclusion

Commercial surrogacy, arising in the late 1970s, began to solidify as a market generating high revenue in the mid- to late 1990s once success rates with IVF increased. As this chapter has shown, today the commercial surrogacy market is dominated by for-profit agencies that peddle a particular framing of surrogacy—heartwarming, safe, and binding—to increase their client base, legitimize surrogacy, and protect their programs from scrutiny.

Surrogacy market players attempt to frame surrogacy as a legitimate and morally sound practice by normalizing surrogacy, which they do by calling on ideologies of genetic kinship through the specific set of surrogacy rules set out in this chapter. Through impression management (Goffman 1959), agencies attempt to present surrogacy as a legitimate and wholesome route to parenthood—one that pulls on the heartstrings. That translates into agencies carefully choosing with whom to work by weeding out undesirable surrogate applicants and choosing deserving IPs. The IPs must be worthy of these services, as indicated by their reasons for pursuing this route to a child. Surrogates must appear to be givers, with pure hearts and clean pasts. They must be mothers who are not motivated by money alone and who think of their surrogacy efforts as their jobs (taking surrogacy seriously and complying with instructions) but not as work (they must see surrogacy as heartwarming caregiving, not a source of profit). All of the parties must appear to be above reproach, because surrogacy continues to be contentious and debated within society. Anything less might spell a media disaster for agencies—another Baby M case. Selecting high-quality surrogates (who will be compliant) and truly needy IPs (who will be grateful) is an attempt to protect agencies and REs from the possibility of having a litigious situation on their hands.

The rules about surrogacy are directly shaped by the bad press that surrogacy has received—recall the assertion of Cheryl Woodley that her agency can't "touch" welfare recipients because doing so would open it up to being "attacked" for doing so "by female libbers." Avoiding bad press goes hand in hand with wanting to avoid court cases. It is here that the shaky legal ground of surrogacy is problematic for the market. The neoliberal orientation of the market allows for a range of services to be available at market-set prices. However, many surrogacy professionals with whom I spoke advocated for tighter regulation of surrogacy (with the caveat that they would prefer to be involved in writing the rules). With regulation, they told me, comes licensing procedures, and with licensing comes state legitimation and the safety it provides. Unscrupulous surrogacy agencies and brokers would be closed or unable to operate freely if surrogacy were regulated by the state—a move that would be welcomed by many of the larger, established agencies. As James Ianson, who runs a surrogacy program as part of his law practice, told me, regulation would "be the death knell for the ding-dong surrogacy agency that's working out of somebody's house and the person is matching because she was a surrogate." Licensed agencies, on the other hand, would be run by professionals—lawyers, psychologists, and social workers—and would receive implicit state support. With legitimate arrangements run by licensed agencies, participants in my study told me, surrogacy would no longer be viewed as transgressive, and therefore their agencies would be safer from public condemnation. The number of scandals would decrease with regulation, and though the gray market for babies might shrink, more people might become interested in surrogacy as a route to parenthood, thus expanding the market. However, the federal government has made no efforts to regulate surrogacy, so market players—agency directors, REs, and attorneys—attempt to police the practice themselves through establishing rules about who gets to participate.

The contemporary surrogacy industry walks a fine line between expanding and increasing its profitability, on the one hand, and remaining culturally palatable by fitting into cultural norms about family reproduction, on the other hand. The development of IVF was crucial for balancing these twin market demands, for it is not only a highly profitable medical procedure, creating a huge market and attracting new industry players, but it also allows for a reiteration of genetic kinship ties that fits nicely with normative ideologies of the family in the United States. Traditional surrogacy, in which the surrogate used her own egg, challenged these basic normative ideas popular in the United States that equate true parenthood with genetic lineage (Jacobson 2008). With IVF, that challenge is eliminated as both intended fathers and intended mothers are able to enact genetic parenthood.

With the move from artificial insemination to IVF, the surrogate moved from the true genetic mother parting with her child (as critics contend) to the woman "merely" providing the womb for gestation for the "true parents." With this realignment of surrogacy with traditional notions of true parenthood, IVF offers the surrogacy market a level of protection from conflict and potential litigation that was not possible with traditional surrogacy. In fact, today some surrogacy market players will work only in the gestational surrogacy realm, avoiding traditional surrogacy arrangements completely. Some REs, for example, work only with gestational surrogates. When I asked Randall Blackborne, the RE, if this was the case with his clinic, he replied:

> Oh yes, absolutely. That's pretty severely frowned upon, [surrogates] using their own eggs. Just for many reasons, but the biggest issue is: who are the actual parents? And if the woman carrying the baby is also the biologic mother, then there's always potential for a conflict later on as to whose child is this? And of course, we want to avoid that at all costs. So that's not typically done very often. I've never done it. I would never do something like that. . . . Others might consider that. Other people probably do that without any medical supervision too. But just not something we're involved in.

Although there are REs, as Randall implies, who do work with traditional surrogates, those who have established clinic-specific rules not to work with such women, such as he has, do so to avoid the conflict that is possible when it is not culturally clear who the actual parents are in a surrogacy arrangement. So although this self-imposed rule limits the market, it is seen to be valuable in terms of the relative safety it provides from litigation over genetic parentage.

The use of IVF alone, however, is not enough to protect surrogacy from scrutiny and litigation. The commercialization of reproduction and babies and the huge profits involved are culturally problematic for surrogacy. As this chapter has discussed, the market attempts to ensure that surrogacy is palatable through a careful selection of participants: the deserving IPs who want genetically related children and, most important, the giving women who act as surrogates. Doing so aligns surrogacy with traditional notions of genetic parenthood and nonmarket feminine caregiving and sacrifice (Folbre 2001). By encouraging this particular framing of surrogacy—altruistic caregiving rather than crass greed— the surrogacy market works to obscure the profit motive. And doing that makes surrogacy more palatable, which in turn ironically makes it more profitable. As the next chapter shows, however, it is not only the selection of IPs and surrogates that is crucial for surrogacy's success. So is a careful socialization and monitoring of surrogates' interpretations of the work in which they are engaging that ensures the profitability side of surrogacy is largely obscured—that surrogacy is seen not as a labor for profit, but as a labor of love.

CHAPTER 3

Laboring to Conceive

SURROGACY AS WORK

I first met Amber Castillo seven weeks after she had given birth to a little girl—
her first surro-baby—via cesarean section (C-section). My jaw was on the floor
as I watched Amber dash around her living room in rural central Texas, taking
care of her two young children and playing hostess to the visiting researcher.
When I made the original appointment with Amber I had not realized she had
had major abdominal surgery so recently, but Amber told me not to worry,
she had quick recoveries. Following all three of her C-sections (two with her
own children in her early and mid-twenties, and one with the surrogacy at
the age of twenty-eight), she was up and about within days. She let me know,
for example, that she had given birth to her surro-baby on a Saturday, and by
Monday she was out shopping (albeit slowly) at Walmart for groceries with a
friend. She also returned to work full time that week. She runs a day-care center
in her home, taking care of two—sometimes three—children, in addition to her
own two during the day. The day-care children were back in her home for full-
time care the same week she gave birth. "Not a problem," she told me, "I just used
a stepstool to help them in and out of their high chairs and their beds. Other
than that, it was absolutely fine."

Quick recovery was one of the reasons Amber thought she would make a
good candidate for surrogacy. Pregnancy, birth, and recovery were not hard for
her—even with the surgeries; they were, in fact, easy and joyful. She loved being
pregnant, she told me, and saw surrogacy as a way to enjoy gestation and birth
without—and this was important—having a new baby to care for in the family.
She did not want another baby; she just wanted another pregnancy. Her family
was complete, and though she wanted no more children, she enjoyed pregnancy
so much that she wanted to experience it again. When she saw an ad for a surrogacy agency in a shopping flyer, something "clicked" and she said to herself,
"I have to do this!"

44

Though I was impressed by Amber's quick, energetic recovery, after time spent in the field I came to see how normal this was in the world of surrogacy. A refrain I heard many times was first shared with me by Treena Winmer, who had been a surrogate twice (both times with twins) in her mid- and late thirties, when she told me, "I carry very easily. It's very easy on me. I don't get sick, I don't ache. And I recover very easily." As a group, surrogates are skilled at pregnancy and birth—and they speak about pregnancy and birth as skills. Pregnancy and birth, participants in my study told me, were processes to be enjoyed and savored, a skill set that could be honed and practiced, and an entity in and of itself—not only a process that produces a baby, but an experience to be treasured. This is why Amber and many of the other women in my study initially saw themselves as ideal candidates for surrogacy: they possess the necessary skill set and they enjoy using it—more than enjoy it, they told me they love it.

When I talk about my research and say that surrogates actually enjoy their surrogacy experiences, my listeners often express shock. The most common responses I receive are "Why on earth would someone want to be a surrogate?" and "I could never do that!" Surrogates tell me that they frequently receive such comments as well, from strangers, acquaintances, and sometimes friends and family members. Sherry Woods, for example, a one-time surrogate in her late thirties who was trying to match with a second set of intended parents (IPs) for another journey, explained that while she was pregnant with her first surro-baby and went out in public, she would get negative feedback from people who knew her situation. She explained: "I got a lot of the whole 'How can you just give away a baby?' crap—or 'give away *your* baby.' It's not mine to give away, so *not a problem*. But I did get quite a bit of that. Or the whole 'Well, I think it's great that people can do that, but *I* couldn't.' That kind of thing. I did get quite a bit of that. And whenever they say that—'It's great that *you* can, but *I* could never give up a baby'—it always implies somehow that you're cold, it really does."

I see three basic assumptions driving the chilly reaction described by Sherry. The first is the assumption that surrogates are parting with their own children. As I will show in this chapter, this is a common conception surrogates confront. The second assumption is the idea that pregnancy and birth hold no pleasure in and of themselves and are painful, unpleasant experiences best avoided—unless you *really* want a baby. With these two assumptions, surrogacy is framed as both morally suspect and illogical. This brings us to the third assumption: that people do not engage in painful, immoral behavior for the benefit of others unless they are immoral themselves or are pressured to do so. Surrogacy only makes sense, from this perspective, if women are coerced into surrogacy by their own greed (or others') or by their own desperate needs.

The image of surrogates that these assumptions evoke is of women somehow lost (or "cold," as Sherry put it), unmoored from what is seen to be the natural relationship between women and the children they bear, coerced by financial reasons to behave unnaturally. Surrogacy challenges basic cultural ideologies of motherhood—those deeply held, socially constructed cultural beliefs that women are the mothers of the children they gestate, that women bond deeply with their gestating babies and newborns, and that women who birth children want to mother them. This idealized model of mothering, popular since the early twentieth century and continuing to intensify (but seen to be "natural, universal, and unchanging") places "responsibility for mothering . . . almost exclusively on one woman (the biological mother), for whom it constitutes the primary if not sole mission during the child's formative years" (Glenn 1994, 3; see also Hays 1996). Surrogacy deeply challenges these notions. With gestational surrogacy, the concept of a unified mother (genetic, gestational, and social) is parceled into distinct and separate bodies, identities, and relationships: three possible women (egg donor, gestational carrier, and intended mother), three bodies, three relationships to the fetus or child (Hartouni 1997; Teman 2010). With commercial surrogacy, not only is reproduction separated from sexual intercourse, but also the act of carrying a pregnancy and birthing a child is divorced from the intimacy of the family and placed within the market. Commercial surrogates are paid to gestate and bear babies and not bond with them in what is thought to be a "motherly way," to not see themselves as the mothers of those infants, and to not engage in the infants' social mothering.

The movement of reproduction into the market and the commercialization of mothering activities have raised deep social, legal, and ethical concerns about surrogacy for the last four decades. These concerns are reflected in court cases, media stories, and public opinion on surrogacy. Surveys since the 1980s have consistently found that most people do not approve of surrogacy, finding it the least acceptable route to family expansion (Dunn et al. 1988; Edelmann 2004; Krishnan 1994; Poote and van den Akker 2009; Weiss 1992). Media stories reflect this repulsion and frame surrogacy as freakish and unnatural, intending to provoke scorn and outrage about these arrangements.

As I explore in this chapter, in public presentations of surrogacy, we can see an intense anxiety about women who engage in third-party pregnancy. Part of this anxiety is about how to delineate exactly what surrogates are doing and why they are doing it. When a woman gestates and bears a child for a family member without pay, that gesture is often framed not as labor, but as a gift given out of familial love. But when a woman makes such an arrangement with strangers for pay—and does it again and again—that labor has the potential to blur the culturally constructed boundaries between work and family. When pregnancy becomes something akin to employment, do families become work?

In this chapter, I also explore how women come to work in the highly contentious field of surrogacy, both the initial seed of inspiration and the motivations that draw them to this practice. I am centrally interested in how surrogates think about the labor in which they engage: Do they consider it employment?

Moreover, how do the negative images of surrogacy shape how they think about their work and the interactions they have with others? How do they negotiate the negative cultural discourse around the commodification of their labor? In exploring the process through which women become surrogates and analyzing the ways in which surrogates talk about their work, I examine how surrogates confront and negotiate assumptions about surrogacy and the negative image of their work. In doing so, I describe the actual labor involved in surrogacy and contemplate links between surrogacy and other forms of feminized labor in the United States.

Surrogate Sample

For this project I interviewed thirty-one surrogates who resided in Texas or California. Two participants had not yet given birth to a surro-baby, though they had a total of seven failed transfers, a miscarriage, and a stillbirth between them. Failed transfers and complications were not uncommon among my sample, nor are they uncommon for in vitro fertilization (IVF) attempts and IVF pregnancies in general (Becker 2000, 92; Katz et al. 2002). Most surrogates had experienced a failed transfer, a chemical pregnancy, a blighted ovum (when an embryo does not develop inside a gestational sac), or a miscarriage sometime during the process of attempting surrogacy. The remaining twenty-nine participants had completed at least one successful surrogacy (that is, a journey that ends in the birth of a live infant): fifteen had completed one journey, seven had completed two journeys, five had completed three journeys, one woman had completed four, and one had completed five. In total, there were fifty-three successful surrogacies among these twenty-nine women that had resulted in the birth of seventy children (twenty-nine singleton births, nineteen sets of twins, and one set of triplets). As my sample attests, the rates of multiples are increased with IVF (Evans et al. 2004; Katz et al. 2002).

Except for the woman who had completed five journeys, women at all other stages were contemplating or engaged in additional surrogacies. Some of my participants had already been matched with new IPs, some were pregnant with additional surro-babies, and others were beginning a new journey. From time spent in the field I learned that repeat surrogacies, as I will discuss in greater length in this chapter, appear to be typical and, if the first journey was a smooth one (in terms of an uncomplicated pregnancy and social relations), successive journeys are encouraged by agencies.

There were certain demographic characteristics that could be found across my sample. Twenty-eight of the women identified themselves as non-Hispanic Caucasian, two as Hispanic, and one as African American. Due to the fact that statistics on surrogacy are not kept, it is impossible to know how representative this sample is of the racial diversity of surrogates in the United States. However, surrogates and surrogate professionals in my study and other researchers have noted that the field of surrogacy in the United States—both in terms of surrogates and of intended mothers—is largely the terrain of white women (Braverman and Corson 1992). Despite early warnings that surrogacy could result in the exploitation of women of color (see, for example, Corea 1985), this appears not to be the case—at least in the United States. The racial homogeneity of surrogacy is consistent with that of assisted reproductive technologies as a whole in the United States (Becker 2000; Bell 2009; D. Roberts 1997).

Like most women in the United States, the majority of surrogates in my sample had worked outside of the home at some point in their lives (only three had never done so), largely in female-dominated professions: teaching, child care, nursing, retail, social work, and clerical work (Bureau of Labor Statistics 2013). During their tenures as surrogates many continued to work, either full time (fourteen) or part time (five), in similar professions—though several now work in various aspects of the nonmedical side of the surrogacy business (as coordinators, recruiters, and agency owners), which is also female dominated. Among the twelve women who were not working at the time of our interview, three were actively looking for outside employment, while nine characterized themselves as stay-at-home mothers. Seven of the thirty-one women had never attended college, though they all had a high school diploma or a general educational development (GED) certificate. The rest had either attended and not completed college (eleven) or had an associate's degree (two), a bachelor's degree (seven), or a graduate degree (four).

None of the women in my sample lived below the federal poverty line, nor did any receive federal welfare aid—a condition, as discussed in the previous chapter, most agencies require surrogates to meet. Nine women in my sample had annual household incomes of under $50,000 per year, while four women had incomes of over $150,000; most of my participants fell somewhere in between. Based on education, occupation, income, and residence neighborhood, I characterize roughly half my sample as working class or lower middle class and roughly half as solidly middle class. I characterize one family as professional middle class.[1]

Eighty-four percent of the women in my sample identified themselves as religious. Catholics and several mainline Protestant groups (Mormon, Lutheran, Baptist, and Methodist) were represented. The largest religious group, however, was "Christian," which tends to denote nondenominational, evangelically oriented groups in these women's regions.

All of the surrogates in my study were mothers. As discussed in the previous chapter, surrogacy agencies have a strict requirement that women employed as surrogates must have birthed and mothered at least one child. Most of the women in my study (twenty-three) had two or three children, though five had only one child, two had four children, and one had five. The average age at first birth was twenty-two—though there was a range. One-third of my sample gave birth to their first child as a teenager (ages seventeen through nineteen), another third between the ages of twenty and twenty-three, and the final third between the ages of twenty-four and thirty-four. Two-thirds of my sample had their first child several years before the national norm, which is currently 25.6 years of age (Martin et al. 2013).

The majority of the women in my sample gave birth to their children within a heterosexual legal marriage. At the time of my first interview with them, twenty-six were married, one was cohabiting with a new boyfriend, one was divorced, and three were single. None of the women in my sample identified herself as lesbian, though I did not ask specific questions about sexual orientation. All spoke of current or former male sexual partners.

At the time of my first interview with them, the surrogates in my study ranged in age from twenty-four to forty-five, with an average age of thirty-four. The average age at first surrogate birth for my sample was thirty-one, though again there was a range. The youngest age at first surrogacy birth was twenty-four, and the oldest was forty. Most had given birth to their first surro-baby in their early thirties, though one-third had been in their mid-twenties, and five had been between thirty-five and forty. The ability of older women to serve as surrogates today (compared to traditional surrogates in earlier decades) can be explained by the fact that gestational surrogates do not contribute their own eggs in the creation of the children. Because uteruses do not age in the way that eggs do, it is possible for women to be surrogates into later life (Abdalla et al. 1997; Bahn et al. 2010).

NEGATIVE DEPICTIONS

In Margaret Atwood's 1987 dystopian surrogacy novel *The Handmaid's Tale*, the US government has been overthrown by a military dictatorship, which quickly revokes the civil rights of women. Fertility is in drastic decline, and there are two classes of women: one privileged to mother and one forced to breed in the context of enslavement, devoid of civil rights, and the ability to have a family life of one's own. I first read *The Handmaid's Tale* in the early 1990s and remember well the feeling of outrage it evoked. Much of the attention given to surrogacy, both by academics and in popular culture, attempts to evoke a similar horrified response. This can be seen in the rhetoric used in surrogacy presentations (for example, wombs for rent), in the visual images that accompany many news stories (such as a pregnant belly surrounded by cash or with a bar code stamped across it), and in the sheer attention given to this route to family formation.

Susan Markens (2007) argues that the intense interest in surrogacy over the course of the past several decades is indicative of the ways in which surrogacy has been constructed as a social problem. Despite its being a rather small social phenomenon, during the past three decades there have been over 6,500 articles in US newspapers and wire services on surrogacy, and much of the coverage has been negative.[2] Surrogacy has been the topic of several films, miniseries, story lines in television shows, and documentaries. Magazines and online media sources routinely have stories about surrogacy, especially as more celebrities make public their use of third-party reproduction.

Some media presentations of surrogacy are saccharine melodramas, such as those found on the Lifetime channel, with positive depictions of surrogates. These stories tug on the heartstrings as they take the viewer through the dramatic highs and lows of third-party pregnancy. Often, the surrogate in the story is a relative of the intended mother and refuses compensation. This is the case, for example, in the 1993 Lifetime movie *Labor of Love: The Ann Schweitzer Story*, starring Ann Jillian, in which the surrogate lovingly gestates and births her own grandchild. In many media presentations, however, surrogates are portrayed as uncooperative, unstable, and desperate for money. IPs are often portrayed as rich, insensitive, and desperate for a biological child. These combined negative character traits are often juxtaposed. For example, accompanying a 2008 *New York Times Magazine* article titled "Her Body, My Baby" were two images: one of the white surrogate, barefoot and nine months pregnant, sitting on the small porch of what appears to be her lower-middle-class home; the other of the white intended mother holding the baby on the manicured lawn of what appears to be her much larger and much more expensive home, complete with a uniformed black baby nurse standing at attention. Judging from the four hundred readers' comments, the images in this story—like *The Handmaid's Tale*—evoked outrage at the assumed economic coercion of the surrogate and the privileged entitlement of the intended mother. In fictional accounts, these archetypes are further intensified for dramatic effect. For example, in the Tina Fey and Amy Poehler comedy *Baby Mama*, the surrogate is not only desperate for money and vulnerable in an unstable relationship with a loutish boyfriend, but also greedy enough that she lies to the intended mother about having achieved pregnancy. And in one episode of the less-well-known *Outer Limits* television show titled "The Surrogate," the surrogacy procedure is not only strange but otherworldly, as it turns the surrogate into an actual alien.

Both nonfictional and fictional media presentations of surrogacy rely on the same archetypal images of surrogates, IPs, and surrogacy professionals to draw interest and solidify particular framings of surrogacy. By "framing," I am referring to the way the media choose to whittle an often complex phenomenon down to a highly digestible and easily recognized, often singular, idea or image (see Jacobson 2014). The hook in both fictional and nonfictional framings of surrogacy is often exploitation. Though members of the general public know little about actual surrogacy, its legality or history, and the intricacies of the related medical procedures, they do understand the concept of exploitation and greed. Many stories on surrogacy, therefore, use easily recognizable caricatures that symbolize an exploitative relationship to explain surrogacy: the victimized infertile woman versus the swindler; the privileged, entitled, upper-class woman obsessed with a genetic child versus the poor baby machine forced to breed to feed her own children. As I will explore further in the following chapter, this can especially be seen in presentations on contemporary surrogacy abroad, in places like India and Thailand, where poor women are impregnated with the embryos of wealthy couples (both domestic and foreign) and kept in hostels for the duration of their pregnancies so that they can be "not just monitored but also controlled" (Pande 2010a).

These archetypes cast surrogates negatively as workers: either they are capitalizing on their fertility to swindle as much money as possible out of vulnerable IPs, or they are forced by the larger structural forces of poverty and gender inequality to capitalize on their reproductive abilities to feed their own children. How do surrogates deal with these insinuations about their character? How do women who are contemplating surrogacy react to these assumptions? Through my interviews, it became clear to me that surrogates are aware of these negative images and work hard to dispel them. As this chapter explains, they largely do so by attempting to undermine the three popular assumptions of surrogates discussed above: (1) the assumption that they are parting with their own children; (2) the idea that pregnancy and birth hold no pleasure in and of themselves and are painful, unpleasant experiences best avoided—unless you really want a baby or are desperate for money; and (3) people do not engage in painful, immoral behavior for the benefit of others unless they are greedy or pressured to do. The pushback against these assumptions begins early in the career of a surrogate and can be seen in the ways in which women frame their initial motivations to engage in third-party pregnancy.

THE INITIAL SEED

When I asked surrogates what initially led them to the idea of surrogacy, I received a variety of answers. Roughly one-fifth of my sample mentioned a surrogacy-related made-for-television movie (often on the Lifetime channel, like the Ann Jillian movie discussed above) or news story (often on the television shows *Dateline* or *Oprah*) that initially interested them in surrogacy. When the women saw these media representations, they felt a connection to surrogacy. For some, this occurred when they were young. Nicole Parish, for example, was twelve when she watched a Lifetime movie about surrogacy with her grandmother. Afterward, Nicole told her grandmother, "I think that's neat, and someday I'm going to do that." From that point forward, Nicole, who went on to become a surrogate at the age of thirty, told me that the idea of being a surrogate "was just always in the back of my head, that I would have babies for somebody that couldn't." When I asked Nicole what interested her in the idea of surrogacy after watching the film, she replied: "I just thought it was neat. I just thought it was something to do for somebody that couldn't do it for themselves. And I've always been a baby person. I mean I started babysitting when I was ten. So I've always been around little kids and babies, and I think babies are neat! So at that age I was just like, 'Why wouldn't you? Why wouldn't you help somebody else if you could? And wouldn't that be like the neatest thing?' And I just carried it with me." The idea of surrogacy being "neat" and something one should engage in if one could was a common refrain of surrogates. Like Nicole, others framed surrogacy as simply helping others in need and incorporated that idea into their life plans from an early age. This was the case with Vanessa Moreno, whose own mother was a traditional surrogate when Vanessa was a child. Vanessa, now in her mid-thirties, had such a positive experience with her mother's surrogacy that from that point forward, she incorporated the idea of surrogacy into her plans for her life's trajectory, even vetting her future husband on the issue.

In contrast to women like Vanessa and Nicole, who thought of themselves as future surrogates from a young age, several women in my sample did not think about surrogacy until it was recommended to them by others due to their ease with pregnancy and birth. For example, Deidre Richards let me know that it was her husband who first planted the idea in her head after the birth of her son, Trevor, when she was thirty-one: "Honestly, it was kind of a joke. After Trevor was born—I had such a great pregnancy with him and I loved being pregnant. And we kind of joked about it. Like three days after he was born, my husband said, 'That was so—you did that so well, and you're so good at carrying babies, you should think about being a surrogate.' And it was kind of a joke between us. But I thought about it and I thought, 'You know what? I think I really want to check into that.'" Surrogacy was suggested to several other women in my study after their family members or friends saw how well they carried and birthed their own children. These women did not indicate that they were pressured to become surrogates by their husbands or family members, but rather that they became intrigued by the idea after it was suggested to them.

Three women began to think about surrogacy after unsolicited interactions with surrogacy agencies. Josephine Maselli received an e-mail from an agency via a post she listed on Craigslist looking for babysitting work. Though she was offended by the solicitation, after a friend urged her to consider surrogacy (based on how well Josephine's own pregnancies had gone), Josephine began to think about it. The two other women who were recruited had first contacted or worked for egg-donation agencies. One of them, Leah Spalding, found egg donation when searching the Internet for ways for "women to make quick money" when she was in her early twenties. She did not find the experience satisfying, however, as she preferred to have a personal relationship with the IPs—which is unusual with egg donation (Almeling 2011). Years later, a discussion with a friend about her egg-donation experience led to a conversation with a mutual acquaintance who was a coordinator at a surrogacy agency. Leah told me that when she learned the details of the surrogacy program, "immediately I was like [snaps fingers], 'I'm ready.' Because you get to meet the parents, you build relationships, and you get to keep in touch with them afterward and I was like, 'I am all over this. This is going to be amazing.'"

In contrast to these positive experiences, which interested some women in surrogacy, three women in my study came to surrogacy via a personal traumatic life event, such as infertility or rape. After having endured those experiences and going on to have children of their own and a happy family life, these women desired to "give back" out of gratitude for having survived. To these women, surrogacy was a meaningful way to "repay" their karmic debts and "rebalance the universe."

The most popular reason, however, for a woman having her interest sparked in surrogacy was witnessing the pain of a family member, friend, or co-worker who had experienced infertility issues. This drew one-third of my sample to surrogacy. For example, Cherise Armstrong, a nurse and three-time surrogate, was first approached by her mother to carry for her younger sister. Cherise, then in her mid-twenties and a mother of two, immediately answered in the affirmative, explaining: "I was like, 'Oh yeah, no problem.' Because pregnancy is pretty easy for me—unlike [for] my mom—and so I said, 'Well yeah, of course. It's my sister.'" In the end, Cherise's sister was able to achieve pregnancy herself utilizing the drug Clomid. The experience of volunteering to be her sister's surrogate, however, and the information about surrogacy Cherise obtained while researching the process, intrigued her. She and her husband continued to research surrogacy, and they decided: "This is kind of awesome. Let's do this for someone." This was a common experience among the women in my sample. Only one of the women in my sample carried for a family member or a friend whom she had known before working as a surrogate for that person. However, for one-third of my sample, the process of volunteering or considering carrying a child for a family member or friend was the event that brought the idea of surrogacy into their lives. Like Cherise, after initially committing themselves to helping a loved one and researching surrogacy to prepare themselves for the process, these women came to see surrogacy as something that they wanted to engage in—regardless of the fact that their IPs would be strangers.

Growing Motivations

As discussed here, there were a variety of reasons why women began to think about surrogacy as something in which they would like to engage. Regardless of the initial seed that planted the idea of surrogacy in their lives, however, there was a common triggering event that propelled my participants to move to action, shifting from thinking about surrogacy to going online and filling out an application. This event was the birth of what they understood to be their last child. Most surrogacy agencies prefer to work with women who have completed their families. The women in my study understood this early in the process and waited to pursue surrogacy until their families were complete. Most women described feeling sad when they realized that they did not want more children (or that circumstances kept them from having more children) and that they would never experience pregnancy and birth again. Kelly Russo, a thirty-seven-year-old one-time surrogate who had been matched with new IPs at our interview, told me that she "loved being pregnant" and that, when she was pregnant with her daughter in her early thirties, she "actually did not want it to end, and when the doctor said, 'I think she's going to come a week or two early,' I said, 'No! I'm not ready! I don't want this to end.' It was like, sad. I was happy to have her but it was sad that stage was over." When I asked Kelly why she was sad, she answered, "I really liked feeling the baby move. I liked the doctor's appointments. I liked everything about it. The whole thing was fun to me. I like the attention of it. Everybody walks by my desk and gets my water for me! [laughs] My big belly. There wasn't anything that I didn't like about it."

All my participants described pregnancy in similar ways to Kelly: they loved the feeling of movement from the developing fetus, they loved their "baby bumps," they loved the attention from others, and they loved how pregnancy made them feel. They spoke of being "energized" when pregnant. Erin Peters, a thirty-year-old three-time surrogate who was on her fourth journey, told me: "I loved being pregnant. I think it's just a beautiful thing. I'm always energetic, and I just love life at that time. And I don't really have a hard time with being pregnant at all. It was easy."

The idea of pregnancy being easy and enjoyable is counterintuitive to popular cultural ideas about the pregnant state. Images on TV and in films of pregnancy feature out-of-control women overwhelmed by their bulging stomachs, afflicted with aches and pains, demanding their husbands to get them ice cream and pickles in the middle of the night, and screaming in childbirth (Morris and McInerney 2010). A common narrative, based on the experiences of many pregnant American women—who undergo some of the highest rates of medical management of pregnancy and birth in the world—is also one of disempowerment, pain, and trauma (Davis-Floyd 2004). In contrast, surrogates reported that they loved pregnancy and when they realized they would never have the opportunity to experience it again, they were "heartbroken." Some said—tongue in cheek—that they were "pregnancy obsessed" and did not know what to do once they were done having their children. Surrogacy provided an answer: they could enjoy pregnancy but not have a new baby for whom they would have to care.

Surrogates not only enjoy the bodily and social process of gestating and giving birth, but they also appear to deeply identify with their roles as mothers. When I met this group of women, I found them to be strongly focused on children. They emphasized the importance of their children in their own lives, and they felt sympathy for people who want to parent but who are unable to have children. This can be seen in the comments made by Andrea Tyson, a thirty-one-year-old three-time surrogate, when she described her reaction to hearing and reading about the plight of IPs:

> You hear these stories that are just so heartbreaking about these people that all they want in life is to have their children and to have their family, and they can't. No matter what they do, they cannot do it on their own. And just to be able to think that I could bring that joy into somebody else's life, especially after having my son—because that changes everything. Every holiday is ten times better. Every day waking up and just seeing that little smiling face or hearing that voice say, "Mommy" or "I love you." There's nothing like it.

The love Andrea has for her son, she told me, propelled her to think, "I can do this for someone." She went on:

> I've always been one of those people that want to somehow help somebody, do something for somebody else. And I just thought, "I'm capable of doing this and I have the ability. Why not? Why not?" And especially at the time I was single. I wasn't having any more children of my own, and I thought, "Why not? Why not help somebody?" And the stories you read online of people, just what they've been through and the struggles they've had and miscarriages. And it's very emotional. And that's where I just thought, "Why not?"

Andrea's phrase "Why not?" was one I heard throughout my interviews with surrogates. It was often preceded by a heartfelt description of the joy of children and words of sympathy for IPs. This was a dominant theme in my interview with Josephine Maselli. As Josephine recounted how she and husband came to the decision to pursue surrogacy, her three young children cycled in and out of the room. We played restaurant with them, "sipping" from wooden cups and "eating" plastic steaks and donuts, as Josephine told me how she and her husband, both in their late twenties, imagined what life would have been like without them:

> We imagined ourselves at fifty, if we had never been able to have children, and you know there are some people [for whom] that would be fine. But for us, personally, never having children or grandchildren to look forward to, nothing—that would be devastating for us. And that was ultimately why we decided we would do this. We knew that if we were in this kind of situation that we would really want somebody to help us. . . . And for us—you know we're Christians, and another belief that we have is that God blesses people individually with different blessings with the expectation that you then share them. That some people are blessed with a lot of money and that He hopes you share that by donating and doing stuff like that. Well, He blessed us with the

physical ability for myself, the emotional ability for our family, and the life circumstances that we could do this. So it just—for us it is kind of a no-brainer. If
I can, why not? So that's kind of what ultimately brought us to where we are at.

Like Andrea and Josephine, most participants framed surrogacy as a
"no-brainer." They possessed these particular skills of worry-free and easy
pregnancies and births, and because they wanted to help others who did not,
there was no reason why they should not become surrogates. For some of the
more religious members of my sample, such as Josephine, ease of pregnancy
and birthing were God-given skills. They therefore felt compelled to share their
blessings with the less fortunate. The importance of children and family, and
what they saw as the desperate need of IPs, overrode any reservations they had
about the surrogacy process. This is what they told me, and this is the dominant
narrative that the surrogacy industry conveys: surrogates engage in surrogacy
because they are good at it, they want to help, and they enjoy it. Tina Vargas put
it succinctly as a "win-win situation": "I just thought, 'Man, I love being pregnant
and there's people who are out there [who want a baby].' And I know adoption
is an option, but there are just some people that really had that desire to have
their own child. So it just seemed to be a win-win situation. I was getting to
fulfill—it was like, 'I can do that well. I can carry a baby obviously well.' So it was
something, not a hobby, but something that I enjoyed doing even as a sacrifice."

DEALING WITH THE PUBLIC

Though surrogates framed surrogacy as a "no-brainer," they noted that they
often encountered people who were resistant to third-party pregnancy because
they did not understand the medical processes involved in gestational surrogacy.
This largely took the form of people assuming that surrogates had sexual intercourse with someone else's husband or that they were artificially inseminated
with someone's sperm and were, therefore, parting with their own genetic and
biological children. Jessica Klein, a thirty-year-old one-time surrogate to twins,
noted that "the first thing" that strangers think about her when they learn that
she is a surrogate is "Oh wow! Her husband is going to let her sleep with that
man?" Jessica explained her reaction to that assumption:

> And I'm thinking, "What's wrong with you? Did you ever think of the first
> test-tube baby?" Let it click there. Put those links together. But people don't
> know. I don't mind educating people. Anybody who asks, I'll tell them, "Ask
> whatever you want. I don't mind answering. I'd rather you ask a weird question
> and I may not answer it than you go around thinking that I'm sleeping with
> some other man. Or that it's my baby and I'm just giving it away." I love to
> answer, and I think that people need to be educated because it is something
> that our world is doing.

Like Jessica, many women told me that they engage in mini-education sessions with their family members, friends, and strangers they meet in public to contradict the negative assumptions about them. Often this begins with basic lessons in biology to correct misunderstandings of surrogacy procedures. Rosalyn Whelan, a twenty-five-year-old new surrogate who had had her first embryo transfer the day before we met, told me that when it becomes known that she is a surrogate, the response is generally, "What are you talking about!?" Therefore, she said, "You have to explain IVF to them. A lot of people don't even understand the process of getting pregnant. And so I've had a lot of *really* long conversations with people."

Rosalyn's statement is telling. According to the National Science Foundation, "many citizens do not have a firm grasp of basic scientific facts and concepts" (2004). Less than 30 percent of the US population is thought to be "scientifically literate," with the majority of the public displaying a "profound ignorance of, and often misinformation about, matters biological" (Klymkowsky et al. 2003, 156; see also Michigan State University 2007).

Surrogates confront this ignorance about reproduction, IVF, and advanced medical procedures when their surrogate status becomes known. They spend a good deal of energy dispelling the misunderstanding that they are the genetic mother (through either sexual intercourse or artificial insemination) of the surro-baby they are carrying. They do so by using the language of biology and genetics, emphasizing that the babies are not theirs because they do not contribute their own eggs in the process. Surrogates told me that the concept of third-party reproduction—that women can gestate fetuses without contributing their own eggs—was new to many people. Because of this, surrogates often use basic language when explaining the medical process. Jessica Klein, for example, would tell people, "I'm basically just the oven. . . . So you just take her egg, his sperm, make the baby in the lab, and there you go. It's very simple."

Many other women in my study also referred to themselves as "just the oven." In doing so, they reinforced the privileged status of biological connectedness between genetic parents and children. So while on the surface, surrogacy might appear to transgress the notion of the "traditional family," in many ways it actually reinforces it. In fact, many gestational surrogates told me in no uncertain terms that they could never act as a traditional surrogate, because that *would be* giving away their children. Dawn Rudge, a thirty-six-year-old two-time surrogate, explained it this way:

> I would never be a traditional surrogate. I would never use my own eggs. I can separate actually having a child for somebody else, because it's not my genetic makeup. You still have the same attachments as you would to your own child when you carry, or at least some of them. But actually having a child with my own eggs—it's too much a part for me. (A) I don't have very good eggs (part

of my medical issues). But (B) I wouldn't do it anyway because that would be a piece of me out there in the world and to me—I can't. Some people can be egg donors and donate their eggs. And some people can carry. And some people can do neither. But I can separate off "this is not physically mine" versus if it's my egg, that's really half my child. So no, I couldn't do that.

Like Dawn, many of the women in my study were aligned philosophically with those people who initially criticized them for "giving away their babies" in that they, too, were averse to traditional surrogacy for themselves, although not for others if they chose to do so. For gestational surrogates, the issue then was one of correcting the misassumption that they were traditional surrogates. Rhonda Chapman, who was forty years old when she gave birth on her only surrogacy journey, for example, told me that when she was discussing her role as a surrogate with others, she found herself specifying that she was a gestational, not a traditional, surrogate:

> When I'd tell people that I was a surrogate, I just felt the need to specify because I felt they might [think I was a traditional surrogate]. And not that I think there would have been anything wrong with it if it were my egg. But again it's one of those things that it's got to be your own personal boundaries . . . you have to know that when the time comes that you're not going to have a hard time separating. And I knew carrying babies that were not genetically related to me, I would not have a hard time separating. A baby that was genetically related to me, I think I might have a hard time separating. . . . And again I never felt like I was giving up babies. I was giving them back. If it were genetically mine, I think I might feel like I was giving it up.

This notion of giving the babies back rather than giving the babies up is an important distinction in surrogacy. Surrogates merely "take care" of the IPs' babies during the prebirth period and "return them" to their rightful parents after birth, I was told. For gestational surrogates, this concept is neatly aligned with popular understandings that privilege genetic parentage. While there is a wide range of family forms in the United States, including various routes to parenthood (for example, genetic, adoption, gamete donation, and fostering), genetic relatedness is idealized as the purest, most natural form (Coontz 1992; Jacobson 2008; Smith 1993). Therefore, many surrogates in my study reported that they challenged criticism not by arguing for the validity of all forms of surrogacy, but by relying on notions of genetic parenthood to support the morality of gestational arrangements. And by and large, this argument was successful for them, as they found that once they explained IVF and the fact that as gestational surrogates they did not share a genetic link with the embryos, fetuses, or babies, people were much more likely to accept them and surrogacy.

The assumption that surrogates are parting with their own children is often coupled with the assumption that they are being coerced to do so by desperation or greed for money. This is a more challenging criticism for surrogates, because most do profit monetarily. The surrogates in my study made between $10,000 and $50,000 per surrogacy journey; most averaged $25,000–$30,000. Those on the higher end of the pay scale tended to be experienced surrogates. These women had successfully completed at least one journey and tended to make more because they had proven themselves and were seen to possess a wealth of knowledge about the process that they could use and pass onto their IPs. Surrogacy agencies directors like to work with experienced surrogates, I was told, because they are "known quantities" and need less guidance and hand-holding than first-time surrogates. IPs like experienced surrogates because of the feeling of safety they generate—and IPs are willing to pay more for that reassurance (Berkowitz and Marsiglio 2007).

During my time in the field, surrogates expressed conflicting feelings about money. Our discussions of compensation often began with the judgment that they felt others made. Sherry Woods explained that there was "a misconception a lot of times about the women that do surrogacy. The whole 'They're bored, they need the money.' Sometimes that's true, but not always. Sometimes it's just the average Jane out there. . . . It's not all a bunch of dummies that are being conned into this and being taken advantage of, like the media likes [sic] to portray." Like Sherry, other women were concerned about the negative portrayal of surrogates in the media and how they have shaped people's understandings of the work surrogates do and the type of people they are.

Surrogates shared several strategies for dealing with criticisms about the compensation they receive. The first was to minimize or hide the amount of their payments. Tina Vargas, a married stay-at-home mother of four children and two-time surrogate in her late thirties who was in the process of being matched with a third couple, told me that when she is asked how much she has been paid, instead of "giving people a number," she replies, "Well, it usually ends up being what a part-time job would be for a year." She does so, she told me, "so that it doesn't really sound like a lot of money. When you get it in a lump sum it does, but if you're talking about no vacation, no sick days, no days off, nothing for a year, a part-time job—then it doesn't really sound as much." Others, such as Allison Farro, a one-time surrogate in her early thirties, noted that "if you add up all the hours, [surrogates are] working for less than minimum wage for what [we] get paid."

Notice that Tina and Allison used the language of work ("no vacation, no sick days, no days off," "part-time job," and "minimum wage") when dealing with criticisms about compensation. This was a common tactic. In doing so, surrogates communicated the idea that surrogacy is work, but not very well paid work. This counters the idea of surrogates as greedily exploiting their reproductive abilities for money. Just as many people misunderstand gestational surrogacy, believing all surrogates to be the genetic mothers of their surro-babies, women told me that people also misunderstand compensation, thinking that conniving women are renting out their wombs to the highest bidders, receiving $100,000 in fees. Gillian Dorsey, in her mid-thirties, characterized it as "a real shame" that people "are ignorant in the world" and think that surrogates are simply a "bunch of welfare moms sitting at home making a buck, pimping out their uterus[es]."

Downplaying compensation allows surrogates to distance themselves from that negative image and to present a more positive framing of their motivations: one based on altruism and gift giving, rather than money making—and one that acknowledges the labor involved but does not frame that labor as a route to quick money. Surrogates took pains to explain that surrogacy does not happen quickly, and that one can be "at work" for years, like Molly Hughes, who was profiled at the beginning of chapter 1, without receiving compensation. In fact, a common refrain I heard from surrogates was that no amount of money alone could motivate one to act as a surrogate. Deanna Meer, a two-time surrogate in her mid-thirties, for example, insisted that surrogacy does not pay well enough to justify being in it just for the money. "It's not about the money," Deanna told me. "They couldn't pay you enough to have a baby for somebody else, at least not me. That's not how it works. It has to be a gift from the heart. It is meant out of love and out of kindness, not for the compensation you get." This is an important distinction in the rhetoric surrounding surrogacy—that these arrangements are not entered into because of financial need or monetary greed but out of desire to help others. Surrogates receive negative press about their labor, and I found most of the women to be careful to avoid any hint of monetary greed. They spoke, as Sherry Woods did, about the financial framing of surrogacy as painful. Sherry said: "It's really hurtful—like people will come on the message boards and call us money-grubbing uterine whores. Like they think that we just do this for money. And it's like, 'No, when you factor in the amount of money that you make for how long this takes, it's like no! No one does this for money.' This is something so life changing that I don't think people understand how much goes into it." Surrogates avoid framing their labor as motivated by money because this would reduce it to reproductive exploitation or baby selling and give opponents fodder for criticism. As discussed in the previous chapter, agencies are careful to avoid surrogates who appear to be "money hungry." As Vanessa Moreno said, money "corrupts" purer motivations: "I don't like it when people ask me, 'How much are you getting paid?' I'm like, it is so not about the money. But you can't do it without money. It's such an emotional and selfless experience that if you tarnish it with just getting money, it's that—it's going to corrupt the whole process."

Vanessa's remark highlights a common belief, that money perverts the purer motivations of surrogates. Similar arguments are made in other contexts, such as volunteerism and gift giving (Titmuss 1997). Interestingly, however, Vanessa is not calling for women to act as surrogates for free. That, she argues, is not possible: "You can't do it without money." There are women, however, who do engage in surrogacy without compensation—known in the surrogacy world as altruistic surrogates. But many surrogates, including Vanessa, argue that such behavior is not realistic. Gillian Dorsey, for example, told me that sometimes women who are thinking about becoming a surrogate "come in there [to an agency] and they're like, 'Oh I'm not doing this for the money, so I want $5,000.'" She went on:

> And every single surrogate who has been a surrogate is going to tell you, "You're an idiot! Your time is worth more than that. What if you're on bed rest? What if you need child care? What if you lose your uterus? What if you die?" These are all valid things. You have to take your own personal worth and decide what it is worth. And how is it going to benefit my family? Because I have small children. They might as well get something out of it. I would probably do it for free because I like to be pregnant, I like to be able to help people, I love to be able to say I'm a surrogate and have everybody say, "Oh you're so wonderful." That's nice. But my kids, they don't get, "Wow, you're so wonderful because your mom's a surrogate." They get a car so that I can drive them to school! So everything that I do, it's for them. And yes, it benefits me, it benefits my family, but anybody who spends five minutes with a surrogate is going to know that it's not about the money. The money is just kind of like a reward for helping. But it's not the be-all, end-all.

Gillian's comment highlights the second strategy women engaged in to counter the negative public image of surrogates: emphasizing the amount of work they engage in, the amount of risk they take in completing that work, and how compensation is a "reward" or insurance policy of sorts for their family. And this is the rub: surrogates want others to understand how much work they do and to agree that they should be compensated for that work; however, many do not want to think about surrogacy as work, nor do they want to openly discuss their compensation or have it questioned. And when they encounter women thinking about surrogacy who they feel do not properly understand the relationship between surrogacy labor and compensation, they are quick, as Gillian says, to "educate" them.

Many participants in my study alluded to bad surrogates: women who were only in it for the money. Leah Spalding, for example, who initially looked into egg donation to make some quick money, told me that she often gets asked about surrogacy by others who "are financially driven." She told me: "They want the money. I've never once met a person . . . who wants to do this just because they are helping someone or because they value family and they believe that everyone should have what some people can't have, you know?" It "took time" for her to learn that:

> Surrogacy is really stressful and hard on your body, and you have to deal with a lot of things. [Therefore] this is something that you should want to do because you want to help someone or because you value certain things. Not because of the money. Because—you might never know. You might go through the whole process and it might fail, and you don't get any money. And then where are you? Nothing [*sic*]. You'll go through your whole life thinking, "Ah, I went through all that for nothing." You know what I mean? When someone else who is doing this for a better reason would say, "Well, we tried, you know. And I really wanted to help you, and I'm so sorry I couldn't." You know what I mean? There's a huge difference. . . . When you are not thinking about the money, you can really open your eyes to what's really going on in the bigger picture.

Just like Leah, Allison Farro spoke about a personal conversion, in which she moved from focusing on the monetary rewards, when "the biggest motivator was money," to concentrating on more intrinsic rewards. Leah, Allison, and other women in my study discussed how that conversion from thinking of surrogacy as a way to make a quick buck to focusing on the gift-giving nature of these arrangements occurred through the lessons they learned being surrogates and through the socialization efforts of the surrogacy community. They quickly learned that if they wanted to be successful in the field of surrogacy and have repeat journeys, it was important to apply the narrative of altruism.

Just as agencies try to weed out women interested only in compensation, surrogates attempt to educate women about the proper attitude toward money—or, at least, the proper way to express one's interests—via online exchanges on surrogacy listservs, in person with other surrogates at social gatherings, and in discussions at agency support groups. As I found in my interviews, the obscuring of surrogacy as work is important to the surrogacy community.

SURROGACY AS WORK

While some surrogates, like Leah and Allison, were forthright about their changing feelings toward compensation, I found talking with surrogates about the work of surrogacy—about surrogacy as work—was tricky. I learned this quickly during my period of data collection. In one of my early interviews, Rosalyn Whelan, a single stay-at-home mother in her mid-twenties who was living with her parents, told me that she "didn't necessarily take offense," but that "most surrogates—if you call it a job, they just get very, very angry, very upset. Or if you call them a professional surrogate, they say 'no, this isn't a job.' They don't want to be considered an employee, they want to be considered like a friend or like a partner." Surrogates are not official employees of either their agencies or their IPs. This is explicitly written into the contracts of many surrogate arrangements. Some surrogates report and pay taxes on their compensation, but based on what I learned in the field, it appears that most do not. This is one of the gray areas of surrogacy. Alexander Franklin, a lawyer in my study who worked with IPs and surrogates, shared with me his understanding of surrogates as independent contractors performing services when I asked him if he thought surrogates were—in legal terms—engaging in work:

> I think that they are being compensated for services, and I think that it's taxable. But there are lawyers who believe it's a gift. I don't know. A gift has to have no quid pro quo, and since you've got thirty pages of contract and money, I'm not sure how you reach "gift." But there are other rationales—that it's some sort of prebirth child support, which legally doesn't exist in Texas. But if it did, I guess you could claim that. I'm not sure. But I don't believe that they fall within, say—like workman's comp[ensation], that sort of employment. But I would think to the extent that you're doing something and you're being paid for it, I would say, yes. Whatever would normally occur in that kind of relationship— yeah, that's employment. Now it may not be wage employment, like when you have a salary or are being paid on an hourly basis or something, but yes, you are providing services and you're being compensated for those services.

Though Alexander discounted surrogacy as "prebirth child care" (particularly in Texas), this phrase came up often in my interviews with surrogates. This phrase is indicative of the ideological knot of contemporary surrogacy that is the focus of this book: when discussing surrogacy as work, I am not talking about legal paid employment, but the contested ideological terrain of how surrogacy is both experienced and framed. Is it exploitation of reproductive capabilities for monetary gain, a gift, an altruistic sacrifice (giving a baby away or giving a baby back), labor, or a hobby?

Though surrogates are not categorized as legal employees (in the workers' compensation sense that Alexander used), the experience of surrogacy is like paid employment in many ways. One of the most striking ways is in the amount of labor and the time it requires. Surrogates in the United States engage in a tremendous amount of work—much more so than with a pregnancy in which one births a child for oneself without the assistance of advanced reproductive technologies. Part of surrogate work is physical, involving medical evaluations and procedures as well as the corporeal process of gestation and birth. Most surrogates undergo a battery of tests prior to being approved by a reproductive endocrinologist (RE) to work as a surrogate and another whole set of tests and procedures during the various stages of a surrogacy journey (cycling on medication, embryo transfer, pregnancy, and birth). Because gestational surrogacies rely on IVF, surrogates must inject themselves (or be injected by

others—most often, their husbands or partners) with the medications necessary for successful implantation and so their bodies do not reject the embryo
or, later, the fetus. These injections range from tiny pricks like people with
diabetes commonly have to shots from large-gauge needles of progesterone in
oil (which can result in painful lumps). Accompanying this medication is not
only physical discomfort, but also mental worry over success. Some—but not
many—women also expressed concern about the long-term effects of taking
this medication.

Part of surrogate labor is temporal, involving the management of a complex
medical protocol and numerous medical visits. Surrogates are often under the
care of several physicians, such as an RE and an obstetrician-gynecologist (OB/
GYN). Sometimes they must also see a perinatologist (an obstetrician special-
izing in high-risk pregnancies), due to the gametes being used. All of these
physicians require screenings, office visits, tests, and monitoring. Managing
their schedules for doctor's appointments, medication, and testing—as well as
ensuring that they kept those appointments, took the medication, and had the
tests—was time consuming for surrogates.

Surrogates also reported that they spent a considerable amount of time
engaging in online research about the processes, medical procedures, and
problems or issues involved in surrogacy. This aspect of their work involves
researching surrogacy and learning from other more experienced surrogates via
online support forums, blogs, and personal exchanges about how to advocate for
themselves and their IPs.

Surrogate labor can also involve a good deal of travel. Some surrogates live
in the same locale as their IPs and use local physicians. Others travel for visits
with IPs (if both parties desire such visits) and for medical appointments. If
medical travel is required, it often occurs at the beginning of surrogacy journeys: to visit the surrogacy agency, to have psychological screening, and to have
medical screening at the RE's office. REs were commonly selected by the IPs
(before beginning the surrogacy process, many IPs had been patients of the RE
they selected), so often those offices were located in major metropolitan areas
convenient to the IPs. Often surrogates have to travel, some by air, to those
appointments and for the embryo transfers. Once surrogates reached eight to
twelve weeks' gestation and the pregnancy was thought to be fully stabilized, surrogates were released into the care of an OB/GYN. Most women indicated that
the OB/GYN who oversaw their surrogacy pregnancies was near to their homes
(often the OB/GYN who had delivered their own children, but sometimes a new
physician they or their IPs selected).

Other aspects of surrogate labor are social, involving what Arlie Hochschild
calls "emotional labor" (1983, 7). As I will discuss in chapter 4, surrogates often
work hard to cultivate certain relationships with their IPs, which involves managing their own emotions. They must also manage relationships between their

family members and those of their IPs; this is part of negotiating work-family balance within their own households and will be explored in chapter 5.

Surrogates told me that they are not "mere vessels," passively being impregnated and lying around gestating their surro-babies. They play an active role in the management and the corporeal process of their surrogacy journeys. The work of surrogacy takes time and energy—which is subtracted from time with their own children and husbands, or partners. Surrogates in my study spoke of surrogacy as "all-encompassing." Using the language of work when telling me about those demands, Tina Vargas said: "You really have to have the right motivation because there's no sick days, there's no days off. It's 24/7 once you get pregnant." She added: "Then just all the shots and the medicines. People are really counting on you, and you can't be flaky about taking your medicines." In the fact that people are depending on you to complete your work, surrogacy is again like employment. For example, Vanessa Moreno, a married part-time office worker with three children, spoke about others' depending on her to successfully complete all of the tasks associated with surrogacy. After two unsuccessful transfers with a couple, Vanessa was getting ready for a third attempt. She spoke of how important it was for her to do her part well, so this couple could have their child:

> It's just like this other family have put the rest of their life, their money, their emotions, and whatever into this. I kind of like have more to think about it. You just have to take it seriously. You just have to think, "This is my job. I have to make sure I take my meds. I have to make sure I stay healthy and eat right. And be more careful in this pregnancy than I have before." Like, I am careful but, I don't know, just a little more careful because this—you are carrying this precious cargo. It's not that it's more stressful 'cause I don't like to have stress, but I think there's a little more riding on it, 'cause you have so many more people involved. So you just have to have the mind-set and the focus and follow directions, like, this is my job and take it serious[ly].

Most of the women in my study took their surrogacy work seriously. The agencies did as well, and this shaped the experience women had working as surrogates. Surrogates speak of working for agencies, though they are not legal employees. They speak of being monitored, in a worklike sense, by agency employees. They speak of needing to "toe the line" and of the possibility of "getting fired" if they do not. They speak of the sacrifices they make to abide by the requirements of surrogacy: especially their medical protocols and doctor's appointments. For example, Kelly Russo shared with me how surrogacy dictated how she spent her time, which made it feel like a job: "I don't want to say I feel like an employee because I don't look at it that way. I hate whenever you see or I read things where the parents are treating the surrogate like an employee. And that's just not a good relationship to have with each other. But it is a job. I have to commit to being at my doctor's appointments, taking my medicine, taking my vitamins. There's a lot of times when I couldn't go do something because I had to have a shot at this time."

Those sacrifices are part of what makes surrogacy like work. Laurel Molza, a four-time surrogate who gave birth to five surro-babies over the course of her thirties, concurred: "You hate to call it a job, but it's part of the job sometimes. You make those sacrifices." It is not only the surrogates who sacrifice time and the ability to participate in regular activities, but, as I will discuss in chapter 5, their children and husbands as well. Surrogacy, they contend, "takes over" their family life because it takes over their lives. Surrogates spoke a good deal about the sacrifices their husbands and children make for them to engage in surrogacy. Deanna Meer, who had been on four surrogacy journeys (two resulting in successful births) for three different couples, contextualized her decision to "retire" from surrogacy by speaking of the physical demands of pregnancy and the time needed for surrogacy: "It consumes your life, it really does. I wouldn't change it, I love it, but it does, it consumes your life. Which is another reason why this is the last one. My husband said, 'Could I have my wife back?'"

Though surrogacy mirrors paid employment in its time demands, responsibilities, pressures to perform, monitoring by supervisors, and work-family conflict, women told me that they did not like to think of surrogacy as work. In making the argument that they are not motivated by money, surrogates argue that financial need is not present, as would be the case in a normal work situation. For example, though Amber Castillo spoke about the financial constraints her family faces, she told me that it was important both to her and to her husband that she not feel pressured into surrogacy:

> We wanted to do it. Financially we did not need to do it. Of course we put the money to good use, but we never let—like my husband said, "If you think you have to do this to make ends meet, just know that's not [the case]." And I said, "No. Of course the money will help, but it kind of takes honestly a couple of years off of the whole plan." Because we sat down, and we have a financial plan. "But I don't feel like it's a job." And that's what he told me, "I don't want you to feel like this is another job that you have to do."

This was an important factor to most of my participants—the idea that they didn't need to do this work, but that they wanted to do it. For most of these women, then, work is something that you do not want to do, but something financial need forces you into. Molly Hughes expressed this view when she told me that surrogacy is not a job

> because I don't have to do it. I want to do this. There are not many jobs out there where I think people would go through this much for a job! I mean this is very emotionally taxing, physically and mentally. And I'm doing it all because I want to. I think it's a job in the aspect of how much time it takes, and

you get compensated. You're doing a job, basically, and getting compensated. I don't *feel* like it's a job. No. Because I could quit whenever I wanted to! And I don't know many people who would go through this much for a job. This is more a personal, fulfilling thing that I want to do for someone else.

From Molly's comments, we can see the dominant folk understandings of work: the ideas that work is not enjoyable, not personally fulfilling, is something we must do because of financial need, and is something for which we are monetarily compensated (Damaske 2011; Daniels 1987). Molly and other women in my study argued that surrogacy is not work, therefore, because of the deep pleasure and satisfaction that surrogates derive from it. This speaks, perhaps, to their past dissatisfaction with paid labor. In fact, surrogates derive so much pleasure from surrogacy that many women in my study expressed guilt about receiving compensation. That guilt was exacerbated by the guilt women experienced because surrogacy took them away from their own families. These feelings of guilt are common for women—all women—engaged in paid labor. As Sarah Damaske notes, women "continue to face historically negative moral connotations about women's paid work: staying at home continues to suggest altruism, while working suggests selfishness" (2011, 6).

Surrogacy, the women in my study told me, was a selfish pursuit—done not because of financial need, but out of desire to experience the pleasures of pregnancy again. Surrogates largely justified compensation, therefore, by spending the money they received on their families (especially their own children). Some used it to pay monthly bills or on family vehicles, but many used at least part of the money to splurge on something special for their children—a trip to Disney World, for example, or starting or adding to a college fund. Using the compensation on their families deflects attention from the pleasure surrogates derive and, simultaneously, takes surrogate labor out of the realm of payment for services, turning the compensation into a thank-you gift for sacrifice. And this is ultimately how most surrogates wanted surrogacy framed: as both an enjoyable experience for them and as a sacrifice they and their families make to help others. They wanted their labor acknowledged, but not acknowledged as work. They wanted compensation and argued they deserved it—but they wanted compensation for their sacrifice, not payment for their services or for the baby.

Only one surrogate in my study was doing a surrogacy journey for free—and this was a "sibling project," to give another child to a couple for whom she had already served as a paid surrogate. Even the women who expressed guilt about compensation received payment for subsequent journeys. One of the agencies with whose staff members I spoke actually insisted that their surrogates receive compensation. Women who balked at doing so were encouraged to donate the money to charity or to place the money in an account in their children's names. The psychologist who works with this agency explained that money serves as an important marker of gratitude from IPs to surrogates, performing an important function of mitigating against feelings that might arise in surrogates of having been taken advantage of by their IPs. It becomes problematic if surrogates refuse compensation, therefore, when they become disappointed with their IPs (most surrogates do at some point, the psychologist told me) because they have nothing to show for their hard work. Compensation, therefore, is an essential part of the arrangement—it ensures that women will become surrogates (since most will not do it for free) and, as I will explored in greater detail in later chapters, helps create a reciprocal, rather than a unidirectional, relationship, which enables the smooth functioning of the market.

Agencies are aware, however, that both surrogates and IPs are uncomfortable with the fact that money is changing hands in such an intimate setting. As I will discuss at length in the next chapter, surrogates and IPs are both invested in having cordial relationships with each other. Money can taint those relationships. Many agencies, therefore, act as the middle man between IPs and surrogates, with all money and talk about it filtered through the agency rather than passing directly from the IPs to the surrogate. Agencies filter the money because surrogacy cannot exist—in today's climate—without compensation.

Conclusion

Surrogacy is a contentious politicized issue, with compensation at the core of today's debate. Surrogates no longer part with their genetic children in the process of surrogacy; IVF has allowed the surrogate's eggs to be taken out of the equation. In place of the debate about surrogates parting with genetic children that dominated concerns about surrogacy in the 1980s and 1990s, the chief social issue arising from surrogacy today is the cultural unease with intensified commercialized reproduction. More women are working as surrogates today, they are engaging in more surrogacies, and they are being paid more for their services. There are also more surrogacy professionals (lawyers, doctors, and staff members of surrogacy agencies) making more money is this arena. There is a cultural unease with what is increasingly understood as a surrogacy industry. This unease can be readily seen in the media attention given to surrogates' compensation. Popular images of surrogates have focused on their fees and what they represent: wombs for rent! Surrogates are confronted by the image of the "money-grubbing uterine whore" and are careful to frame their labor in a positive light. They do so by dealing with the three core assumptions about their work and their character: they explain that they are "just the oven" for someone else's "bun"; that they enjoy pregnancy and birth and are quite good at both; and, most important, that they are not desperate for money, forced to be surrogates by poverty, or attempting to capitalize on their fertility at someone else's expense. Rather, they argue that surrogacy is a "win-win situation" in which women skilled at labor and birth and who profoundly enjoy the pregnant state are able to help bring children into the world for people desperate for "their own children." I found the more experienced a surrogate was, in terms of time spent in the reproductive marketplace, the more deeply entrenched she was in the rhetoric that attempts to protect surrogacy from criticism. Protecting surrogacy largely equates to the valorization of surrogate motivations and the erasure of the idea of surrogacy as work that produces monetary gain. Ironically, however, by disallowing a discourse of surrogacy as work, the tremendous amount of labor these women engage in—in other words, their sacrifice—is also obscured.

In the obscuring of surrogate labor, we can make links between surrogacy and other female-dominated occupations. Many women are currently employed doing work that has been traditionally performed without pay by women in the home: looking after children, caring for the elderly, cleaning and cooking, nursing the sick, and educating the young (Duffy 2011). As Susan Reverby (1987) has shown, skills acquired in the home have historically been parlayed into employment by women, especially widows and those who were single for other reasons. Normative ideas about women and work position women as especially good at this type of labor; women are socialized into providing it and are often encouraged to pursue paid work in those fields (Coltrane and Galt 2000; Daniels 1987; England 2005; Fisher 1990). Surrogacy can be seen as fitting within this framework, on this continuum of steady expansion of the market into family life as surrogates gestate and birth children—a primary female activity within families.

The concept of "reproductive labor" is helpful here. Feminists scholars used this term to capture and make visible "women's nonmarket activities—housework, child care, the servicing of men, and the care of the elderly—and [to define] all those activities as *labor*" (di Leonardo 1987, 441; see also DeVault 1991; Hartmann 1976; Oakley 1974). Many scholars today use the term "care work" in place of reproductive labor and have added relational aspects (such as "the activity of attending to others and responding to their emotions and needs" [Coltrane and Galt 2000, 16]) to hands-on care to more fully understand this kind of work. Though there is some variation in how scholars conceptualize care work and some debate about which occupations should be included in this category, interestingly the gestation and birth of children is often not included; the laboring activities listed by many scholars center on the care of people who have already been born. I argue that the work of human reproduction—that is, the gestating and birthing of children—should be seen as a kind of reproductive labor or care work inasmuch as gestating and birthing children is care of children (and of embryos and fetuses), part of the social reproduction of families, and an essential activity for ongoing human existence. World overpopulation aside, as a species, we need children to be born. And in twenty-first-century America, the gestation and birth of children can take considerable mental, physical, and emotional effort.

Those who have studied various forms of care work have shown that women's caring labor is devalued (not seen as real work), as evidenced by low wages and little prestige, which is made possible especially because this labor often occurs in the home or in homelike settings (such as nursing homes) and is therefore often hidden from public view (Abel 2000; Daniels 1987; Fisher 1990; Glenn 1992; MacDonald 2010; Romero 1992). Wages are also kept low because this labor is often framed not as work that requires skill, but as that which makes use of feminine abilities that arise naturally in women (England 2005). Women are seen to be ideally suited for caring work, and the caring occupations are dominated by women (Dodson and Zincavage 2007; Duffy 2005; Folbre 2001).

The notion that women are inherently better at caregiving presupposes that men and women are inherently different. As gender scholars have shown, the idea of essentialized gendered difference creates hierarchies of power and privilege (Hartmann 1981). The gendered division of labor disadvantages women, both in the home and in the workplace (DeVault 1991). Ironically, it is a rhetoric of love and sacrifice—of care—that enables this inequality because it permeates understandings of women's work, allowing low wages, little prestige, and less-than-ideal working conditions. As Pierrette Hondagneu-Sotelo argues in her work on immigrant domestics caring for children in Los Angeles, "parents want someone who will really 'care about' and show preference for their children; yet such personal engagement remains antithetical to how we think about much employment" (2001, 10). Normative ideas about work and family and the divide conceptualized between the two position carework in a liminal state: not quite family love and not quite paid employment. When it comes to caring work, then, wages are kept low because the work is meant to be a calling and done out of love. High wages are seen as representative of noncaring employees—and when care is the service, the use of noncaring employees is seen to equate to lower-quality service. In a capitalistic society in which value is designated monetarily, the low wages in female-dominated occupations are framed as a badge of maternal sacrifice, displaying workers' commitments to care and the way we like to think about that care as genuine, as love. Paula England and Nancy Folbre (1999) write about this as a care penalty. Just as unpaid work in the home is viewed as unskilled drudgery, so, too, is paid care work of a similar nature (Daniels 1987). Caring labor is infused with contradictions: it is given lip service as valuable (at least by those needing it), yet ultimately seen as unskilled; it is culturally valorized, yet not adequately compensated—precisely because it is labor engaged in by women and seen as an expression of inherent female skills, interests, and abilities; work that is hidden because it is family work.

Surrogates frame their work as sacrifice, neatly positioning surrogacy alongside other forms of female-dominated labor. Their work is meant to be a labor of love, arising out of their nature and womanly skills. Of course, while some men have entered other female-dominated fields, especially the older markets of nursing and primary-school education, being a surrogate mother is impossible for men. Because of this, surrogacy is perhaps the most uniquely feminine of all the female-dominated occupations. The rhetoric that undergirds surrogacy—one of self-sacrifice and altruism—is, therefore, inherently gendered, with ideas about women and reproduction used to support the industry. It is a familiar narrative, allowing the system to function.

Like other care workers, surrogates call on the rhetoric of self-sacrifice and love in framing their labor. However, they emphasized that they—and their families—deserve compensation not only because of the time demands involved but also because of the bodily risks they take and the specialized skills they bring to the market. But the intrusion of the market into reproduction that surrogacy represents—the outsourcing of making babies, among our most intimate interactions—provokes general anxiety and, as survey research implies, is repugnant to many (Edelmann 2004; Hochschild 2012; Krishnan 1994; Weiss 1992). This anxiety can be seen in the attention surrogacy garners in the press and in Hollywood, despite the relative low estimated numbers of surrogate births per year. To neutralize that anxiety, the strongest marker of the market, compensation, while essential for the market to operate, needs to be obscured for that market to be culturally palatable. The surrogacy market depends on surrogates; yet, ironically, cultural anxieties about the commodification of reproduction and children have resulted in a marketing and cultural discourse that either largely obscures the actual labor (including the attached compensation) or pathologizes it. Surrogacy in the United States is therefore seldom acknowledged as a legitimate and culturally sanctioned form of paid employment—even, as this chapter has explored, by those engaging in it. The obscuring of surrogacy as work plays out in various dimensions including, as the following chapter shows, the relationships that surrogates in the United States create with their IPs.

CHAPTER 4

Managing Relations

SURROGATES AND THEIR
INTENDED PARENTS

Surrogacy, like medical transplants, plastic surgery, and call centers, has been outsourced to places around the globe with lower overhead costs and less regulation than in the United States, and with large, compliant, and cheaper labor forces. Various arms of the third-party pregnancy industry now operate in countries such as Belarus, India, Mexico, and Thailand and cater to wealthy domestic and international clients. We know the most about surrogacy in India, via both the sparse academic literature on the subject and the higher-profile media stories such as the documentaries *Google Baby* (2009) and *Made in India* (2010), television segments on *Oprah* and the national news, coverage in print or online by publications such as the *New York Times, USA Today*, and the *Washington Post*, and numerous online commentaries on sites such as the *Huffington Post*. Examining what we know about India is helpful for highlighting key aspects of surrogacy in the United States.

We know, for example, that surrogacy is much cheaper in India than it is in the United States: estimates place an Indian surrogacy in the range of $25,000–$40,000, while a US surrogacy can cost three times that amount (DasGupta and Das Dasgupta 2014c; Rudrappa 2012). We know this lower price tag is what primarily draws American clients to seek surrogacy abroad (Shetty 2012).

We also know some details about the structure of surrogacy in India and how it differs from that in the United States. Unlike women in the United States who reside at home and remain (mostly) embedded in their regular day-to-day activities during their time as surrogates, most (but not all) Indian surrogates are housed in hostels run by the clinics for which they work. In these hostels, they are fed, given medicines and vitamins, encouraged to rest, sometimes taught new skills (such as sewing, how to use computers, and English) and closely monitored (Madge 2014; Pande 2014). This housing arrangement helps protect surrogates from discrimination they might otherwise experience due to their participation in this highly stigmatized activity in India (Hochschild 2012; Nayak 2014). Indian surrogates are paid an estimated $2,500–$7,000, a figure that reportedly would take these women decades to earn working outside of surrogacy (DasGupta and Das Dasgupta 2014a; Delhi IVF n.d.; Madge 2014; Pande 2010b, 974; Shetty 2012).

We also know that most Indian surrogates have no or very limited contact with or knowledge about the intended parents (IPs) of the children they carry (Hochschild 2012; Rudrappa 2012). During the surrogacy journey, the information about the pregnancy that IPs receive most often occurs via communication with the clinic, not via surrogates themselves (as is typically the case in the United States). For foreign IPs, part of this is likely due to language and cultural barriers, but there appears to be more involved. Contact between surrogates and IPs is seemingly peripheral to the structure and experience of surrogacy in India. While there is some movement toward contact between Indian surrogates and their IPs (see, for example, Arieff 2012; Bailey 2014), most reports place the clinics as the clear middle men, with direct contact between IPs and surrogates nonexistent or extremely limited. Any contact that does occur is usually arranged and monitored by clinic staff.

The image we have been given of surrogacy in India, therefore, is of a service-sector outsourced labor market (Hochschild 2012). There is no window dressing in the presentation of Indian surrogacy, no obscuring of the labor via the structure of surrogacy arrangements or the framing of this practice by the Indian surrogacy industry or the surrogacy community itself. It is work, the surrogates are workers, and the product is the baby. It is an economic transaction—however, one that is presented by the global media, the Indian surrogacy industry, and the larger surrogacy community as win-win: IPs want children, and Indian surrogates want money. We are told that the compensation Indian surrogates receive enables them to build a house, buy a car, educate their children, or otherwise provide some upward mobility for their families. Poor women are explicitly recruited as surrogates in India, since the payment they receive is thought to potentially be so life-transformative that it justifies women engaging in what is otherwise understood to be a highly stigmatized activity. Therefore, according to this frame, not only does Indian surrogacy enable people to become parents, it empowers poor women in India to change their own lives and the lives of their families (Markens 2012; Nayak 2014). Surrogacy in India is presented as "opportunity, choice, and fair exchange," a way for women to pull their families out of poverty and for infertile people to have their much-desired children (Bailey 2014, 27). At the least it is seen as "mutually advantageous exploitation" (DasGupta and Das Dasgupta 2014a, 180).

Some contest this win-win framing of Indian surrogacy as equally beneficial to both IPs and surrogates. Susan Markens (2012) calls this alternative conceptualization the exploitation/inequality frame. In this framing, it is precisely the economic disparities shaped by the global inequities between clients and surrogates—what enables Indian surrogacy to be framed as win-win—that many in the United States and elsewhere find both problematic and, as evidenced by the explosion in media attention to the subject, fascinating. In this contested framing, Indian surrogacy is possible because of what the anthropologist Shellee Colen calls "stratified reproduction," the ways in which the "bearing, raising, and socializing of children and of creating and maintaining households and people (from infancy to old age) is differentially experienced, valued, and rewarded according to inequalities of access to material and social resources in particular historical and cultural contexts" (1995, 78). In other words, Indian surrogacy is possible because of the economic and global inequalities between Indian surrogates and Western IPs and the different values placed on the creation of both groups' children, their reproductive rights, and the quality of their families' lives. Sayantani DasGupta and Shamita Das Dasgupta argue, for example, that Indian surrogacy is a "progeny of a post-colonial and post-globalized world order" that "privileges Western white parenthood, and specifically Western white maternity, over Indian motherhood" (2014a, 195). Surrogacy further compounds this inequality, according to this contested framing, rather than being an antidote for it.

It is helpful to think about surrogacy in the United States against the backdrop of Indian third-party pregnancy because of their similarities and the different ways they are framed and experienced. Surrogacy in the United States is also framed as win-win by the industry and surrogacy community: IPs want children, and surrogates—what exactly do surrogates in the United States want? Money? Yes, as discussed in the previous chapter, money definitely enables women to work as surrogates in the United States. Though none of my participants identified money as the reason they were surrogates, recall that only one of the women refused compensation. Even so, according to the dominant narrative in the United States, money alone cannot be the primary motivator. Recall in the last chapter how US surrogates told me that there was not enough money to propel anyone to engage in surrogacy. But apparently there is in India. The sentiment of being motivated primarily by money, while it may be felt in the United States, is not acceptable rhetoric in the surrogacy industry or community here in the global North. Remember the market rule discussed in chapter 2, which is common in the United States, of not allowing welfare recipients or otherwise economically unstable women to act as surrogates. In the United States it is seen as problematic to have as surrogates women who are obviously economically vulnerable. The opposite is true in India, where poor women are specifically recruited because of their economic status (DasGupta and Das Dasgupta 2014a).

For surrogacy to be culturally accepted in the United States, it cannot be seen as a blatant exchange of womb for money, as it is presented to us as being seen in India, nor can it even be a primarily economic exchange. Surrogacy in the

United States needs to be framed quite differently—still as win-win, with each party obtaining something of value from the arrangement. For the IPs, the object of value is clear: if all goes well with the embryo transfer and the pregnancy (which is not always the case), they receive a baby. But what do surrogates get? If money is not the primary motivator (as surrogates told me), what is? Outside of the joy of pregnancy, what do women hope to gain from acting as surrogates?

In describing their surrogacy journeys—the choices they made, the advice they would give to others, the disappointments, and the joys—it was clear that the something more beyond compensation that surrogates hope to gain from surrogacy is a particular experience, what many of them referred to as a "perfect journey." Perfect journeys result in live births of babies, of course, but perhaps the most important element in this desired experience is the relationship surrogates cultivate with their IPs. Unlike the situation in India, where the surrogate-IP relationship is limited or nonexistent due to geographic distance, language and cultural barriers, and a particular business model that views the relationship as unnecessary, in the United States the surrogate-IP relationship is central to the structure of surrogacy and the experiences of surrogates, IPs, and surrogacy professionals.

In this chapter, I examine the importance of that central relationship and argue that it operates to help stabilize the industry and make surrogacy culturally palatable. I explore how surrogates and IPs determine what type of relationships they want to have with each other, and how agencies try to facilitate certain types of interactions between the parties. I also use this chapter to examine surrogates' conceptions of themselves, reproduction, and birth and how they are changed through their relationships with IPs and their experiences in the world of surrogacy. I show how the close relationships established between IPs and surrogates function to obscure surrogacy as work. I also analyze the ways that tensions arise in relationships when that labor is not obscured and how distant relationships highlight surrogacy as labor. In doing so, I show how the relationships between surrogates and IPs represent potentially destabilizing elements for the surrogacy industry and, therefore, have to be carefully managed.

First Contact

At the beginning of a new commercial surrogacy journey in the United States, especially for first-timers, the surrogate and the IPs are often strangers to one another. People sometimes meet via online support websites, such as surromomsonline.com (commonly referred to as SMO) or through friends, family members, or acquaintances in the surrogacy community. There is no way to know how many independent (indy) matches occur, just as there is no federal accounting that would enable us to know how many agency matches occur. Two of my participants "went indy" after first having worked for an agency, and another one completed her first journey without an agency. The rest of my participants were introduced to all of their IPs by an agency. Judging both by my interviews with surrogates, surrogacy professionals, and IPs and by the information available online at surrogacy websites and in online blogs, this appears to be a typical experience for commercial surrogates.

While the actual process of matching surrogates and IPs can vary from agency to agency, it is the agencies (rather than the surrogates, the IPs, or the reproductive endocrinologist [RE] clinics) that often manage the selection process. Matching surrogates with IPs is the agencies' primary activity. Larger agencies might hand IPs a large binder of selected profiles or give them a password to an online database and allow them to pick which women they would like to meet. Likewise, some agencies hand surrogates profiles of several different IP clients and ask them to identify the IPs with whom they would like to work. Smaller agencies might present IPs with all of the potential surrogates they have and allow the IPs to select their surrogate. But a more typical process is for the agency to whittle down the number of possibilities and exert more control over who may end up with whom. Sometimes this means allowing IPs to read the profiles of a couple of different surrogates, and sometimes it means presenting the IPs with the one potential match. This is not only more efficient, surrogate professionals told me, but it allows the agency to manage more carefully the matches in an attempt to avoid some of the pitfalls—which will be discussed below—that can occur with what I heard called "bad matches."

In a typical process, a staff member at the agency is charged with matching the parties. Sometimes this staff member is a trained psychologist, other times it is the agency director or surrogacy coordinator (who may or may not have credentialed counseling training or an advanced degree). Before the advent of in vitro fertilization (IVF), when surrogates were the biological mothers of their surro-babies, the matching process was more difficult, as the focus was on matching phenotype and other genetic characteristics (height, for example) between surrogates and intended mothers and in ensuring the egg donor met other criteria of the IPs—often things like an advanced education, athletic ability, and musical aptitude (for criteria typically used for egg donors, see Almeling 2011). Agencies also needed to ensure that surrogates' eggs were what those in the industry refer to as "high-quality eggs" and therefore had stricter rules when it came to the age of their surrogates and their genetic normality. Today, with gestational surrogacy, the surrogate's genetics (in terms of phenotype and age and other characteristics we often mistakenly attribute to genetics, such as musical aptitude) are immaterial. As long as she can sustain a healthy pregnancy and give birth, her race and coloring, age, and eggs are considered irrelevant. This has made the matching process simpler. It is also easier because many more women are eager to act as gestational surrogates, compared to those who were willing to birth genetically related children under traditional surrogacy.

With IVF surrogacy, agencies, especially the large ones, have a much larger pool of surrogates than they did when the only way to be a surrogate was to use your own eggs. The task of matching surrogates with IPs has therefore switched from a focus on genetics to a focus on interpersonal compatibility.

To help determine compatibility, agencies create profiles of IPs and surrogates via a series of questions regarding such things as termination (abortion), selective reduction (of embryos), number of embryos to be transferred, and the amount of contact each party desires both during and after the surrogacy journey.

Surrogacy professionals stressed that it was extremely important from the beginning of the match for the IPs and surrogate to be "on the same page" when it came to the big ethical quandaries. Because of this, some of the larger, more established agencies require counseling or intake sessions with potential surrogates and IPs to work through their feelings about ethical issues that may arise. This doesn't always happen, however. Most of the smaller agencies in my sample did not require this, nor is there any regulation that would require this of those completing an independent arrangement. Alexander Franklin, a lawyer who works with a large surrogacy agency and who also handles the legal paperwork for independent surrogacy arrangements, told me that some of his cases have gone badly due to mismatches between IPs and surrogates on ethical issues:

> I've had independent arrangements where the parties aren't on the same page as far as even the basics of if something was seriously wrong—we'll say amniocentesis showed a serious physiological abnormality of a child, say Down syndrome, something like that. And I have couples saying, "Absolutely, we would want to abort." And then the surrogate is saying, the attorney is coming back and saying, "No. She is just opposed to that morally, religiously, whatever." And that's a problem. That's when I tell the couple, "That's a very basic issue that can happen. It's not some pie in the sky thing. Yeah, it's unlikely that it happens, but you may have a child that has Down syndrome and if you do, how are you going to react to that?" And so, a lot of times, what you'll see is pressure being applied and the surrogate says, "Well, okay. I guess I would consider it." And the couple says, "Okay, deal done." And my reaction is, and I put it in writing, under Texas law, of course, you can't force somebody to make that health decision. That's the surrogate's, she has the right. And I don't know of a court in any other state that I'm familiar with that would force a woman to have an abortion just because the IPs say that's what they want. So those are very tough issues.

Those "tough issues" and the instances in which they have led to litigation serve as cautionary tales to surrogacy professionals. Ensuring good matches is a key industry strategy for avoiding the courtroom. As Alexander said, "the bottom line is you want your surrogate to have the same belief set as your [IP] couple. As long as that's okay, then you're probably 90 percent going to be okay if something bad happens." The key issue here—the "bad" that can happen—is the situation in which a decision about selective reduction or termination needs to be made.

THE BIG MATCHING ISSUES:
SELECTIVE REDUCTION AND TERMINATION

Selective reduction, a process in which one (or more) fetus in a multifetal pregnancy is "eliminated through an injection of potassium chloride, which stops the fetal heart," and termination, in which the entire pregnancy is eliminated, are the most potentially problematic issues in the relationship between surrogates and IPs (Mundy 2007, 253). Some surrogates refused to work with IPs who would consider termination or selective reduction; many more stated that they deferred to the parents. When discussing abortion, Deidre Richards, a two-time surrogate and owner of a small agency, highlighted this dilemma:

> Most intended parents I've worked with want the medical decisions to be left up to them. There are a lot of surrogates that will not terminate or selectively reduce under any circumstances. And so if they're not on board on that issue, then we don't enter that phase or send that profile to [the IPs]. The chances of that having to happen or even coming across that are probably pretty slim. But you don't want to get into a situation where the surrogate says, "Absolutely not. I will not abort this child." And the parents are saying, "This is my child, and we're not going to raise it because of these medical issues or what have you." So there's got to be a compatibility issue that way.

While Deidre and Alexander both remarked that selective reduction and termination are rare, they do occur. One participant in my study, Andrea Tyson, a three-time surrogate who was matched through an agency that exclusively served foreign IP clients, actually found herself in this situation twice. Her experience highlights the importance of the surrogate-IP relationship in the dilemma of selective reduction.

Andrea had already given birth to a singleton for an overseas couple when she was matched with another foreign couple. With this new couple, three embryos were transferred, resulting in a twin pregnancy. Though there were no known abnormalities in either of the fetuses and both were thought to be healthy and developing well, the agency director pressured Andrea and the IPs to consider a reduction from two fetuses to one. Andrea was shocked. Though the Centers for Disease Control and Prevention does not collect data on the number of selective reductions that occur, most reductions are thought to be higher-order births (triplets or quadruplets) being reduced to twins (Centers for Disease Control and Prevention 2011; Mundy 2007, 266). This is what Andrea thought as well.

She had not considered being asked to reduce from two to one. She was not alone in this belief. According to Mark Evans (considered to be a pioneer of fetal procedures, including reduction) and colleagues, "until recently, multifetal reductions to a singleton were rare" (2004, 102).

It is not entirely clear why Andrea's agency director was so set on reduction. His concern seems to have been focused on the additional expenses that could ensue (including caring for Andrea) because of a twin pregnancy. The IP couple was foreign and from a country with socialized medicine. They did not have health insurance in the United States and would have to pay out of pocket for all medical expenses. According to Andrea, the agency director cautioned the IPs that Andrea's health would be at risk with a twin pregnancy. He then stressed to Andrea the financial burden that a twin pregnancy would pose for her IPs should a stay in the neonatal intensive care unit (NICU) be required.

Though the agency director went about pressuring each side to agree to reduction based on how it would negatively affect the other party, because the intended mother (IM) spoke English, she and Andrea were able to communicate directly and learn that each wanted to move forward with the twin pregnancy. The director was not happy, according to Andrea. He even flew them all to Hawaii for a meeting to try to convince them to accept the reduction. Andrea was perplexed: "Here are these people so excited to not get just one baby but two. And I was willing to carry them, so why not?"

The fact that Andrea's IP couple was foreign placed them in a vulnerable position. As they did not speak the language fluently or live in the United States, they did not have access to their own physicians or lawyers but used those secured by the agency. They also were probably not familiar with US laws. Though not illegal, surrogacy is not practiced in their country, nor is it a topic of open social discussion. Information they received about surrogacy was likely funneled through the agency director. The same appeared to be the case for Andrea. Though, of course, she is fluent in the language, she lived at the time in a state that had no surrogacy protection. She was new to surrogacy and was not yet embedded in the surrogacy community, from which she could gain information or perspective. She seemed to rely heavily on her agency for information, guidance, and understanding of surrogacy, her role, and her rights as a surrogate and gestating woman. This may explain the extended negotiation Andrea and her IPs had with the agency director over the selective reduction. Andrea told me that she and her IPs "were finally able to convince the agency director" that they wanted to continue the twin pregnancy, "but it took both us telling him, 'This is what we want to do.' And just being very firm about it." Andrea carried the twins to term.

The story does not end there, however. Andrea's next surrogacy, with the same agency, was a "sibling project" for her first couple, for whom she had already borne a son. She agreed to work with the same agency again because she had developed a close connection to her first IP family and had had a great first journey with them. Two embryos were transferred, which were both graded as low quality. The IPs and Andrea were surprised to find themselves pregnant and even more shocked to discover it was twins. This time, however, the IPs agreed with the agency director that they should reduce to a singleton. Although during the screening and matching phase of the journey Andrea had agreed to selective reduction if so desired by the IPs, she was devastated. And because the IPs did not speak English, Andrea felt she was unable to fully communicate to them that she was willing to carry the twins to term. Andrea was concerned that the director was once again pressuring the couple to reduce by emphasizing the health risks that she herself might face. She even volunteered to take legal responsibility for one of the twins after birth. That idea was quickly rejected. Therefore, she reluctantly agreed to the reduction because, she argued,

> I still feel it's their children, it's their decision. I feel that way. I've felt that way all along. And I agreed to that. I agreed if they chose selective reduction, that's what I would do. But to be honest with you, you don't think you're going to be in that situation and especially twins to one? I absolutely didn't think [that would happen]. And I always thought if there were three and they chose to do selective reduction, my body probably couldn't carry three. So if they chose that, I know that would be the right decision. But I never thought I'd be faced with two to one.

The reduction had a negative impact on Andrea's relationship with the IP couple. While they had been close during their first journey together, which Andrea called "this incredible experience," once they decided to reduce the pregnancy to a singleton, Andrea said, "I just kept thinking, 'How can they choose between these two babies? How can they choose only one?'" And because of this, she went on, "it kind of changed my opinion [of them] a little bit, because I was just shocked that they could do that." Despite how upset Andrea was by the reduction, she carried through with it and then continued the pregnancy of the singleton to term. Because of her experience, Andrea cautioned others, "as a surrogate they always tell you, 'Don't agree to selective reduction if you're not okay with it because it happens.' And I think it happens a lot more than people realize."

It is precisely the kind of situation that Andrea experienced and the potential it holds for a surrogacy journey to sour or fall through completely that shapes the emphasis on screening surrogates to ensure that they will, like Andrea, carry through with their agreements and on making good matches.

Business or Pleasure?

A second major issue in matching surrogates and IPs is the kind of relationship they desire to cultivate with each other. Everyone invested in surrogacy (surrogates, IPs, and surrogacy professionals) desires smooth relations between the parties. Smooth relations not only enable more pleasant interactions, but they also are a buffer against the possibility of litigation and negative media exposure. According to Deidre Richards, the owner of a small surrogacy agency and a two-time surrogate herself, in addition to termination and selective reduction, communication and contact are the big issues when attempting to ensure smooth relations between surrogates and IPs in terms of the desired relationship. "Some intended parents want it to be strictly a business thing," Deidre told me. Their mind-set is: "We're 'hiring' this girl to carry a baby for us. We don't care to get close to her or her family. All we want in the end is our child." This is problematic, Deidre stated, because "most surrogates want more than that. They're doing this because they're touchy-feely people and they want a relationship with the couple! So that can be an issue."

As Deidre indicated, most surrogates chafe at the idea that they are a hired womb. Some agencies coach IPs on this point, teaching them about proper contact and involvement so their surrogates feel supported. But many agencies attempt to avoid this problem from the beginning through the proper matching of surrogates and IPs. Alexander Franklin explained that it can be more complicated than a simple dichotomy of surrogates desiring personal contact and IPs wanting a business relationship. Sometimes, he said, the opposite is true:

> You will have any number of surrogates who say, "I really don't want a lot of contact with the couples. I know what I need to do. I've been pregnant three times before, four times, whatever it is. I've never had any problems with babies. And I'll be polite. I'll do everything I'm supposed to do but I really don't want—this IM is not my best friend. And I don't want that kind of relationship." And then you'll have some surrogates that are saying, "Oh, I want to go out shopping for baby clothes with her. If she has a baby shower, I want to be there." And it's very much of a personal involvement. And so that's the other thing the agency is trying to do. You get an IM that wants that contact and you get a surrogate that doesn't—well, you're going to have a lot of friction. And so you do try and match.

Most surrogates did expect regular contact during the journey with their IPs. For some this took the form of their IPs attending every medical appointment, frequent get-togethers with each of their families, and steady contact via texts, e-mails, phone calls, and Facebook postings. For others, the contact was less intense, but the surrogates felt connected to their IPs. Women who did not experience this, whose IPs looked at their relationship as a business exchange or who had little contact with the surrogate during the pregnancy, felt that something was missing from their journey. This was the case with Erin Peters, who birthed four children for three different couples and had been matched for her fourth journey when I met her. Looking back on her first journey, which occurred when she was twenty-five years old, Erin realized that her match had been less than ideal based on the different perspectives on contact that she and her IPs had:

> I think the first couple, we were just very different. They're very business ori-
> ented and just already have so much stuff going on. They had been through
> surrogacy before, so they probably just were like, "We know what has to be
> done." And I think they were just, "We'll pay you. Okay." Not really worried
> about much else. Just getting the baby and having the means to get that. And
> me going into it without ever having experience or knowing any other surro-
> gates of anything, I guess I was just like, "Well, they seem like good people." I
> wasn't thinking that you need to maybe talk to a few couples before you make
> your decision so you knew that you had a good combination. You know? It
> wasn't like there was anything bad per se, it was just really not fulfilling in
> being [an] "able-to-connect" kind of relationship.

Erin's use of the word "fulfilling" captures a key characteristic of the perfect journey many women were chasing. As Erin noted, she had been at a disadvantage
because she was new to surrogacy and had not yet learned to evaluate couples.
After her first journey, she sought a more fulfilling experience, going on an additional two surrogacy journeys. When choosing her next IPs, Erin was a bit more
discerning, trying to find people who wanted to be involved in the process. This
was something that most of surrogates appreciated. They wanted to enjoy the
pregnancy with their IPs. They also wanted to know that their IPs were going to
make good parents, and one way IPs displayed this was by showing an interest
in the pregnancy and the minutiae of the obstetrician visits by either attending
the appointments, Skyping into them, or calling or texting afterward to find out
what had happened. IPs who had little contact with their surrogate appeared
to be uninterested in the pregnancy, which worried surrogates a great deal. As
Erin's experiences show, finding the right IPs to share a perfect journey can be
a complex process.

GETTING PICKED: THE RIGHT SURROGATE

According to my interviews with surrogates and IPs, the matching process
can feel like dating—especially the modern style of online dating in which
each party sizes the other up via profiles, pictures, and personal testimonials
before deciding if they would like to meet. My interview with Leah Spalding,
a first-time surrogate who had recently been matched with a foreign couple,
demonstrated the jitters that accompany meetings between surrogates and prospective IPs. Leah and I met several weeks before her new IPs were to fly into
the United States to meet her for the first time. Leah had been rejected by an IP
couple in the past and was quite nervous about the meeting. During our lunch,
Leah envisioned what would happen. "When we see each other," she said,

"I'm probably going to start crying, just because of the whole situation. Why are we doing this? I'm not just meeting people. I'm going to be giving birth to their child. So it's like, nervous. Am I going to be good enough? They've seen my profile but they haven't really seen the real me. So I'm really, really nervous." When I told Leah that her IPs were probably nervous as well, she countered, "They're probably not as nervous as me, 'cause I kind of feel like I'm being put on the spot. It's like they're buying a car or something." Leah was excited to have been chosen for a face-to-face get-together but afraid that the IPs might find her unworthy to carry their child. "You don't just choose anybody to have your baby," she noted. "It has to be a person that carries themselves well and is healthy and loves kids and things like that. Not just some bum off the street."

Implicit in Leah's concerns about being considered a "bum off the street" is uneasiness about the differences in social class between her and her potential IPs. Leah was a twenty-six-year-old single mother of two who had briefly been homeless, living in her car, while she completed her associate's degree. Her potential IPs were an older married couple, professionals with advanced degrees and successful careers, who had the means to afford surrogacy. Leah was alert to those differences. They needed her, but would they like her enough to choose her to carry their child? Like Leah, other women told me that they were nervous about the evaluation process of being selected as surrogates. Most were aware that the initial meetings with their potential IPs was a time for the IPs to—using Leah's analogy—kick the tires to see if they want to buy the car and agree to the match. Surrogates were nervous about being evaluated because they understood it was not just their pregnancy and birthing skills that were being appraised (they felt quite confident about those), but their character, lifestyle, and social class indicators and the choices they had made in life. In addition to concerns about health, pregnancy, and childbirth, IPs were generally looking for a surrogate with a stable home life, a supportive environment, someone who they thought was a caring and good mother to her children and who they thought they could trust. Generally seen as problematic were brushes with the police; arrests or convictions for driving under the influence; mental health issues; living in unsanitary housing or dangerous and crime-ridden neighborhoods; histories of recreational drug use or problems with alcohol; being too heavy or too skinny, both of which can make achieving pregnancy difficult; and having partners or former partners who were smokers, unemployed, drug users, involved in criminal activity, and/or imprisoned.

Due to these types of issues, some women are rejected as surrogates by one agency or set of IPs, but accepted by others. For example, Leah had a former partner, the father of one of her children, who was incarcerated. It was for this reason, she had been told, that IPs had rejected her in the past. Though there were years between her and that relationship, she felt she had to manage that issue carefully to demonstrate that she would make a good gestational carrier, that she was not a "bum off the street."

This careful presentation of self was not limited to women like Leah who had potentially problematic issues in their profiles. Rather, when describing the matching process, most of the women could be understood to be engaging in what the sociologist Erving Goffman (1959) calls impression management. They were trying to control the impression that IPs would have of them to demonstrate that they were good people who could be trusted with others' children, despite any differences between them and the IPs in terms of housing, lifestyle, or education. Goffman argues that we all attempt to present our best selves in social situations. The matching process between potential surrogates and IPs is an extended heightened interaction (involving the reading of profiles, selection of certain women, initial phone calls or e-mails, and first face-to-face meeting) in which both parties, like daters, are highly invested in appearing desirable to the other.

One impression management strategy women used to demonstrate their worthiness for being selected as a surrogate was to appear not too demanding when it came to compensation and various other aspects of their contracts. This was the case with Rosalyn Whelan. When I met her, the day after her first embryo transfer, Rosalyn realized that she should have included more fees in her contract and increased her total compensation package. She had not done so because she "kind of felt intimidated. I wasn't really thinking about protecting myself or my family. I was just like, 'Oh, I want them to pick me!'" Rosalyn felt that she "had to win them over" and tried to do so by offering to carry a baby for "a lot lower [fee] than average." Rosalyn felt that this was a way to both increase her desirability to potential IPs because she could save them money and to indicate that compensation was not her primary motivation, thus signaling her altruism.

This strategy was more popular with first-time surrogates who worked for agencies that allowed them to negotiate their fees (some agencies have their own pay scales and do not encourage deviation from them) or who were independent. First-time surrogates are at a disadvantage when they are on the market because they are competing with experienced surrogates. Experienced surrogates not only have what surrogacy professionals call "proven uteruses" and a wealth of knowledge about the surrogacy process, but they have also demonstrated that they abide by their agreements to hand the child over at the end of the journey. Because of this, the base pay for experienced surrogates is usually higher, and many IPs are willing to pay it because of the peace of mind that working with a proven surrogate offers.

The impulse to appear desirable vis-à-vis other potential surrogates (and their lower fees or greater experience, for example) was fed by a discourse of competition and exclusivity in the surrogacy industry. Surrogacy agencies have developed this discourse by cautioning newly enrolled surrogates about the amount of time it can take to be chosen by IPs, which adds to the heightened importance of being selected to talk or meet with IPs. This happened to Molly Hughes, the surrogate profiled at the beginning of chapter 1. She had been told by her agency that "some surrogates have been on the list for two years," waiting for IPs to select them. When her profile was chosen by an IP couple for a phone meeting after only four months, she was elated. "It was down to me and one other surrogate," she told me. Molly spoke with the IM for a good two hours, with the coordinator for the agency listening "quietly in the background." Afterward the coordinator told Molly, "Okay, they really like you. They're going to call this other surrogate, and you should probably have an answer in about two days. Give it three days." However, thirty minutes later the coordinator called and told Molly that she had been selected. Molly was thrilled: "I remember that feeling. It was one of those feelings you don't forget, like the time you were proposed to or the time you found out you were pregnant. It was a big deal!" Many women spoke of feeling a similar euphoria on being selected to serve as surrogates. For example, Gillian Dorsey shared her amazement about being selected. "I feel so honored that they chose me," she said. In addition to Gillian and Molly, other women spoke of the special honor of being selected as a surrogate.

The combination of the excess supply of women eager to act as surrogates, the selectivity used by some agencies in signing surrogates, and the competitive nature of the matching process made me wonder how selective surrogates were about the IPs with whom they chose to work. Did women feel as though they had to accept the first IPs who selected them because they might not get the chance again, or were they more discerning? What I found was that two factors affected surrogates' selectivity: the matching structure in their agency (For example, were they given several IP profiles to consider? Or were only IPs allowed to choose with whom they wanted to work?) and the number of times surrogates had engaged in surrogacy. The more experienced women seemed to be more discerning when it came to selecting IPs, less likely to engage in impression management tactics such as lowering their fees, and more willing to wait for the perfect match. Many were similar to Erin Peters, agreeing on their first journeys to carry a baby for the first IPs who selected them, but becoming more selective on subsequent journeys.

Ironically, just as some agencies caution surrogates they may have a long time to wait until they are selected by IPs, creating a sense of exclusivity, some IPs reported that their agencies communicated a similar sense of urgency and exclusivity in being selected by surrogates. Robin and Gerald Clark, for example, had been told by their agency that "it was very hard to find a surrogate; there weren't enough to go around. It could take years to get one." They were presented with an experienced surrogate, Ann, and the idea communicated to them was: "We found a good match for you because she's too old to be a surrogate; you're too old to be parents. So she'll take you, and you'll probably take her because beggars can't be choosers." Robin was generally pleased with the agency and was new to surrogacy, so she did not know if what the agency was telling her was the truth. However, she said, "because of my feeling of scarcity, we just accepted that," and they went with Ann. Encouraging these feelings of scarcity on the part of IPs and of competition or exclusivity on the part of surrogates can be seen as an industry strategy that helps make matches between parties on the market whom the agencies characterize—as they did Robin, Gerald, and Ann—as less than ideal.

THE BEST IPs

Many women indicated that when evaluating IPs they were looking for a "spark" or a "pull on the heartstrings," language similar to that of falling in love. Others have found this as well in studies of surrogacy (Berend 2012; Ragone 1994). Dawn Rudge, a two-time surrogate and mother of four, used this language when discussing her first meeting with one of her IP couples. "It was just love at first sight," Dawn told me. "I mean, we walked in there and we were all butterflies in the stomach and it was a great match. I don't know how to say it. I couldn't have handpicked a better family." When I asked Dawn what it was about her IPs that made her fall in love with them, she mentioned several characteristics that were commonly desired traits in IPs for the surrogates in my study.

As discussed in chapter 3, for some women the initial motivation that drew them to surrogacy was their relationship with someone struggling with infertility. Though most of the women in my sample did not go on to serve as surrogates for those friends or family members, the idea stuck with them that surrogacy was a way to help others in similar situations. Surrogates desire to work with what they considered to be worthy IPs, those who have a true need for surrogacy. Dawn, for example, was originally drawn to surrogacy because of a friend at work who had cancer. When she met her first IPs, the IM had battled cancer and was seeking a surrogate because of the removal of her uterus. This resonated with Dawn because of her earlier experience with her co-worker.

In addition to true need, many surrogates look for a personality connection or overlaps in character traits between themselves and potential IPs. For example, some surrogates and IPs, especially IMs, share interests or hobbies, and discussing those helps facilitate the initial connections. Erin Peters was impressed that one IM brought a scrapbook to their initial meeting, because Erin also makes scrapbooks. Gillian Dorsey was moved to select her first IPs because she and the IM liked the same TV show. Gillian had been taking her time during the matching process, narrowing down her selections until one day when she and the potential IM were chatting, "she said something about *Grey's Anatomy*, 'That's my favorite show ever.' And I go, 'These are my people!' She's really great. We had all this stuff in common, and then we had the [same] favorite TV show. So that was kind of the point where I decided, 'Okay, these are the people that I'm going to do this for.'" These seemingly small and tangential similarities were imbued with importance for Erin and Gillian as they attempted to make connections with strangers.

However, other surrogates indicated that they had little in common with their IPs outside of surrogacy. Differences in social class played a role in this disconnect. Though there were several surrogates in my sample who indicated that they had similar means as their IPs, most who discussed this topic with me said that their IPs had considerably higher socioeconomic status than they did. It was not unusual for surrogates or their husbands to remark, as Angela Cross—a three-time surrogate in her late thirties—did about one of her IP couples: "They introduced me to a very different lifestyle." Angela's IPs lived "in a huge, giant $10 million house in Beverly Hills," and while they were "not famous, they mingle with famous people," while she lived a solidly middle-class life. The class disparity between surrogate and IP was not that stark with all my participants, but most surrogates indicated that they and their IPs moved in very different social circles. For example, when speaking of one set of IPs, Joel Winmer—whose wife, Treena, was a two-time surrogate—told me that "had we not known them through [surrogacy], we never would have met them. The social circles just would never come together." Others had the same sentiment. Tina Vargas and her husband, Louis, did not originally think that "regular people" hired surrogates, only "rich people." This early belief shaped Tina's interactions at the initial meeting with her first IPs. The IM, Tina told me, "seem[ed] to be very educated, just using all these big words." Neither Tina nor Louis had attended college, and they were concerned that they would not be able to connect with IPs. Differences in social class initially caused hesitation about certain IPs in the selection process for other women as well. April Palmer, a thirty-five-year-old mother of two on her third surrogacy journey, explained that because IPs "have to have money" and are often in a "different class" from surrogates, "you get a little nervous about that." April shared with me the effect of that dynamic on the matching process with one of her IP couples, a couple whom April first rejected based on their profile: "They were just very different from us. Both of them grew up very wealthy, just seemed totally—and their pictures! They looked very—I don't know what the right word is, but not very down to earth. They looked kind of hoity-toity to me. Not snobby because that's not the right word, but maybe a little stiff. And we're really down-to-earth people." April was thirty years old at the time, and she was concerned that the couple, who were considerably older than she and her husband (such an age difference between IPs and surrogates is common), would not like them because of their lower socioeconomic class and younger age. "Are we going to seem young and naive to them?" she wondered. This was a concern that quite a few of the surrogates expressed about their initial meetings with IPs. April's program director convinced her to reconsider the couple and meet them. April agreed and found that she "liked them right away" because "they were really down to earth, and they were not what I expected at all."

Other women who expressed concerns about potential IPs originating in social differences changed their minds about particular couples at the initial meeting during which IPs typically share their painful path to surrogacy. Dawn Rudge, for example, was drawn to her IP couple because during their match meeting the IPs "were very open, very nice, and very much wanted this." Dawn connected with them "immediately," telling me: "I mean, we both cried during the whole meeting because it's emotional. And she brought pictures of their house and their dog. And you just knew it was going to be a good family." It was not only, or even primarily, the ability to provide economically for potential children that surrogates noted as an indicator of a "good family." Rather, regardless of any "hoity-toity" or "rich attitude," it was the intensity of the IPs' desire for a child, shown by their struggles to conceive, that indicated to surrogates that the child would be cared for and loved.

The making of a "good family" and the surrogates' role in that creation were important to the participants in my study. Molly Hughes felt strongly about this: "It helps when I know that this baby I helped bring into the world is going to go off with a family that I trust. And I may not have any place saying that, but I feel within myself if I helped them have a baby that they're going to take care of that baby. And then the baby is going to be raised with good morals and a good family." Molly and other surrogates evaluated IPs in terms of the type of families they were creating. Andrea Tyson, for example, the surrogate who was pressured into selective reduction, had interacted with a potential domestic IP couple whom she later rejected. When they visited her, they told her that they lived in a mobile home without heat, and that their cat frequently brought bats into the house through the cat door. Andrea told me: "I hate to be judgmental. I don't mean to do that, but I just pictured this little baby crawling around this dirty floor and bats coming in the house and no heat. And I'm just thinking, 'I can't do this. I can't be the one to help them.'" Others also rejected potential IPs based on lifestyle. Some surrogates, for example, refused to work with same-sex couples or with single people. Others specifically sought out gay couples, single or older parents, or people they thought other surrogates would reject. The more religious surrogates refused IPs who insisted on retaining the right to terminate or selectively reduce a pregnancy. Others felt strongly that those medical decisions were for the IPs to make—some surrogates, like Andrea, believed this in spite of their own ethical or practical concerns. Some found working with foreign IPs exciting, while others wanted IPs close to home so that they could regularly participate in doctor's visits.

These variations demonstrate that all surrogates do not share a single definition of a "good family" based on lifestyle. The various definitions of a "good family" are consistent with research that shows that increasingly people in the United States "have an expansive definition of what constitutes a family" (Pew Research Center 2010). The diversity in family forms present in the contemporary United States are reflected in surrogates' multiple understandings of what is a "good family" and the political and divisive nature of societal acceptance of that diversity.

Interestingly, however, one criterion I found consistently among the women in my sample, regardless of their stance on other lifestyle issues, was the desire to work with IPs who did not yet have children. The one exception to this was those women who were doing another surrogacy for the same IPs for whom they had already birthed a child (called a "sibling project"). Surrogates told me that they were focused on "creating a family," not just adding another child to a family that already had one. April said: "I was just hoping to help someone who desperately wanted children." This sentiment was especially true for first-time surrogates. Nicole Parish, for example, was initially presented with IPs who already had children. Her boyfriend at the time said: "I thought your goal was to give somebody a baby who didn't have one? The first time you do this, you need to get exactly what you want"—which was to help a childless couple. Nicole eventually selected childless IPs instead.

Surrogates wanted to witness their IPs becoming parents for the first time. They wanted to be the person who enabled the transformation of their IPs from childless couple to family; some even wanted show this off to others in the surrogacy community. This held symbolic meaning for surrogates. Some claimed that childless couples were more attentive IPs. Laurel Molza, a four-time surrogate, noted a difference between her one IP couple that already had a child and her other couples. The IPs with a child "were very nonchalant about the whole thing," she told me. "Apparently . . . they went from [being] like a neurotic with her [their first surrogate] to [being] very absent with me. The things that I always found were really important, like the twenty-week ultrasound and things like that, were kind of lost with them. I always got the attitude, 'Okay. Been there, done that.'" Most women did not want their IPs to have that kind of blasé attitude about their journey. Thus, surrogates often expressed the desire to assist IPs without children in language popular in the surrogacy industry and community of "giving the gift of life" and making their IPs' "dreams come true" by "making families." Results from recent public opinion polls show that many people in the United States believe that it is the presence of children, not just a committed couple, that makes a family (Pew Research Center 2010).

Another important criterion surrogates used for selecting IPs was the desire to work with IPs who used their own gametes and not those of egg or sperm donors. This was something "that was really big" for Amber Castillo and her husband: "We didn't want to do, like, an egg donor. We wanted it to truly be their baby, because we felt like if it wasn't then maybe adoption could be an option for them, because you're still not having your own kid together. . . . So that was really big with us—that it had to be their egg and their sperm, no matter what."

In Amber's comments we can see the ways gestational surrogacy can serve the idea that biological connections between parents and children should be privileged over other routes to parenthood. This belief is not unique to surrogates, of course. Many people in the United States see biology as the standard and preferred route to parenthood (Cahn 2013; M. Nelson et al. 2013). Though there is much variation in family form in the United States, there are a multitude of ways that the hegemonic, heterosexual, nuclear, family is privileged (Jacobson 2008). One way is in the omnipotence of biology, blood, and genetics in the language we use about families. Dorothy Smith (1993) conceptualizes this as an "ideological code," the standard North American family (SNAF), that generates a particular language about families. We can see the SNAF in Amber's comments. She was quite emphatic that the baby she was helping to create needed to be the biological genetic child of her IPs so that it would "truly be their baby." If IPs are not using their own gametes, surrogacy does not make sense to Amber and others who hold this view. Children created using donor gametes, Amber argues, are—like adopted children— not the real children of their parents. It is the sharing of genes and blood that constitutes a true parent-child connection, according to Amber.

Surrogates noted that they found it easier to work with IPs who had a genetic connection with their children. Laurel, who worked both with heterosexual couples who had used egg donors and those who had not, had no qualms about working with those who used donor eggs; however, she found the IMs in those couples to be more difficult:

> With IMs that use egg donors, there are a lot of insecurities because they love this child, they want this child, that child belongs biologically to their husband, but because of their own circumstances that child doesn't biologically belong to them. So I think there's a lot of entitlement issues. And I had that with my second couple. Until she had that baby in her arms, there was just— we kind of walked on eggshells a little bit through the pregnancy just trying to keep her involved and make her feel—kind of held her hand through pretty much the whole pregnancy, just to let her know that, "No, you're not the outsider in this whole experience."

Negotiating the emotional terrain of a nonbiologically related IM was an extra layer of labor for Laurel. The surrogacy community is diverse, however, and there are various routes to the creation of children via surrogacy. Though the community celebrates IVF as a way for IPs to create "their own children" via biological connections, the same community has fashioned a structure and discourse that views the intention to create children as the marker of true parentage when donor gametes are used. There are many IPs who use donor gametes and challenge the idea that they should not be considered the "real parents."[1] Some of these IPs first try surrogacy using their own gametes and, when unsuccessful, go on to use donor eggs or sperm. Some are men with sperm issues or women who do not produce eggs or who produce eggs that are not viable for reproduction. Others are gay men, lesbians, or single people who need to use donor gametes from the beginning of their journeys because they do not have opposite-sex partners.

There are surrogates who are not only willing to help gay men, lesbians, or single people but who prefer to do so. Many of these women see surrogacy as transgressive of conservative notions of the traditional family and celebrate their participation in challenging the status quo. Those who assist gays and lesbians wear rainbow flag T-shirts that say "Surrogate Pride." Some surrogates work exclusively with gay couples, and there are agencies, especially in California, that have programs specifically for gay men.[2] Some women support gay rights and nontraditional routes to parenthood and thus prefer working with gay men. Others work exclusively with men because of what they see as the challenge of working with IMs, who they feel have not emotionally worked through feelings of loss related to infertility. People in the surrogacy community sometimes use the term "womb envy" when referring to this situation.[3] Erin Peters was sensitive to this issue when choosing her second IPs. She rejected one IM because "she still had too much emotional stuff going on." Erin was "very scared that if you go into that, it will be a very big roller-coaster ride of insecurity, her not having dealt with things." Erin chose a different single IM to work with, but other surrogates prefer to avoid the potential for womb envy altogether and work with gay men for whom fertility loss is not necessarily a part of the surrogacy equation.

A final criterion I found that surrogates in my sample used to select IPs was the possibility of establishing a close friendship and having frequent contact with IPs before, during, and after the pregnancy. Surrogates want to enjoy their pregnancies with their IPs. They do not want to be ignored, they told me, "just off gestating someone else's baby" without any attention. Many surrogates want to participate in what they view as the enjoyable aspects of pregnancy, such as shopping for maternity clothing, picture taking, talking about fetal movement together, and attending the baby shower (if invited by their IM to do so). Too little contact denied surrogates the opportunity to witness the joy they were bringing to their IPs. It was important for many of the women to know that they were making a life-changing difference in the lives of their IPs. Most wanted their IPs to come to at least some of the obstetrician visits because it was in those exam rooms where the important moments of surrogacy often occur: the confirmation of pregnancy, hearing the fetal heartbeat, learning the sex, estimating the size, and making decisions. Witnessing their IPs experiencing those moments was important for surrogates. There were some for whom this was not a priority, but many in my study told me they enjoyed this aspect of surrogacy. Many surrogates, therefore, wanted to be matched with IPs who also viewed this type of contact and interaction as important.

The surrogates in my study desired authentic relationships with their IPs, especially their IMs—relationships that were rooted in honest exchanges and open dialogue, ones that "felt natural." This can be seen in the comments of Dawn Rudge. When discussing how she selected her IPs and how she felt about their relationship (which she thought was a good one), she told me that she did not want her IPs to feel beholden to her "just because I delivered their baby." She said: "I didn't want to feel like they were obligated to have a fake relationship with me." Many other surrogates also considered frequent contact and the development of a genuine close relationship that continues after the surrogacy journey has ended to be ideal (Berend 2012). Jessica Klein, a two-time surrogate, who was at the beginning of her second journey when I first met her, expressed this idea: "When you're looking for a surrogate, traditional or gestational, you've got to go in and say, 'We're going to be friends.' And if you can't be friends, I don't think people should work together." She continued: "If you go through all that together, how can you not be friends?" Though Jessica was asking the question rhetorically, many of the relationships between surrogates and IPs were more complicated, sometimes fraught with tension and disagreements. Though everyone involved desires smooth relations and good matches, points of contention do arise.

WHEN THINGS GO BAD

Quite a few of my participants likened surrogacy to a roller-coaster ride, with emotional ups and downs, hormonal twists and curves, and sometimes the bottom dropping out from underneath them. The medical process itself can be intense, especially because the stakes are so high. There are many "hurry up and wait" moments as both parties move from matching through screening and contracts to embryo transfer. Emotions run high at times—especially as people are injecting themselves with large amounts of hormones (and dealing with natural hormonal surges that occur during pregnancy and following birth), large amounts of money are changing hands, and the attempt at pregnancy via surrogacy is imbued with heightened importance as it often represents IPs' "last chance" at genetic parenthood after years on the infertility train. In the midst of all this is a relationship—one that started between strangers—and a contract binding the parties to their obligations and to each other.

Contracts are important tools for establishing the parameters of the arrangement. They contain details about parentage and custody, compensation, agreements over termination and selective reduction, contact, and any stipulations the IPs or surrogate chooses to include (and have approved by the other party), such as conditions regarding food, travel, and birth arrangements. Contracts are powerful tools for compliance (Malhotra and Murnighan 2002). Women often explained their inability to engage in certain types of behavior because of their contract (for example, "I can't travel to see my grandmother now because she lives out of state, and my contract forbids travel after thirty weeks"). Surrogates viewed their contracts as legally binding—and they are for the big issues of parental rights in states in which legislation exists to protect the particular arrangements into which people have entered. In Texas, for example, a legally married couple who contracts with a surrogate and files with the court can have their parental rights enforced by the state if the surrogate attempts to claim custody of the surro-baby. However, in the many states in which the legality of compensated surrogacy has not been tested and no legislation regarding it has been passed, surrogacy contracts are essentially nonbinding (remember that there is no federal protection of surrogacy). In addition, in some states, like Michigan, commercial surrogacy has been tested in the courts and found to be illegal. What this essentially means is that even if a surrogate has a contract in a state that protects surrogacy (or in one in which state-level legality has not yet been tested), she could flee to another state, give birth, and be considered the legal mother of the child. This scenario is rare, but it has occurred and receives a lot of media attention when it does. The Crystal Kelley case—involving the Connecticut surrogate who fled to Michigan after refusing to abort an abnormally developing fetus, as discussed in chapter 2—is the most recent example to hit the national media of a surrogate reneging on her agreement. This scenario, a nightmare for the surrogacy industry, is one of the biggest concerns—perhaps the biggest—for IPs. Because of this very real concern at the center of surrogacy arrangements in the United States, trust is an important element in surrogate-IP relationships.

Both surrogates and IPs spoke often to me about the issue of trust. It was vital in their relationships with each other, they told me, but it did not come easily for everyone involved. There are various risks in surrogacy, for both IPs and surrogates, which some of the participants in my study found challenging to accept. Surrogates had concerns about their treatment at the hands of REs, agencies, and IPs and about their (and their families') relationships with their IPs. They risked being treated poorly, being subjected to unnecessary and painful medical procedures, being left with medical bills, and not receiving their agreed-on compensation. A few—but not many—noted slight anxieties about possible long-term negative heath repercussions from the medications they injected or ingested during the IVF procedures and pregnancy. They worried about medical complications and the impact of multiple births and cesarean sections. Several shared with me their apprehensions about IPs' abiding by their agreements and assuming custody of surro-babies at birth.[4]

Most IPs have experienced previous unsuccessful infertility treatment and heartache in attempting pregnancy, and many feared that their failing streak would continue into surrogacy. Some IPs have difficulty believing that they will achieve parenthood, which leads them to distrust the optimism many

surrogates and professionals display about the process. IPs risk not only failure in pregnancy and continued heartache, but the loss of their considerable
monetary investment should they not achieve a live birth. IPs pay for medical
procedures and associated surrogacy fees whether a child is produced or not.
Satisfaction is not guaranteed in the high-profit world of assisted reproduction.
Most agencies do not require IPs to pay surrogates their full compensation if
the journey is unsuccessful, but the bulk of the fees associated with surrogacy
are due to the agencies, the REs, and the lawyers whether or not a child results.
IPs risk unscrupulous agencies' disappearing with their money—as happened
with the agency SurroGenesis, mentioned in chapter 2 (Federal Bureau of
Investigation 2013a). When IPs discuss their monetary investment in surrogacy,
their concern is not about spending the money to attempt pregnancy per se (and
being unsuccessful). Instead, it is about what the money represents: their ability
to pursue other routes to parenthood, such as egg donation or adoption, should
surrogacy not succeed.

IPs risk their surrogates' being unable to achieve pregnancy because of surrogates' medical issues or misbehavior (for example, failing to take their medicines as directed) or behaving in ways dangerous to the health and safety of their
embryo or fetus. IPs risk their surrogates' refusing to abide by their agreements
on selective reduction, termination, or parental rights. Some IPs fear surrogates
will bond with their babies and refuse to release them following birth.

Some of these trust issues, for both IPs and surrogates, are related to having confidence in their agencies, their REs, and the process of surrogacy, while
others have to do with interpersonal trust between IPs and surrogates. The
organizations involved in surrogacy (agencies, RE practices, and law firms)
have specific methods for fostering consumer (IP) trust through legitimization efforts, including strategies for increasing success in pregnancy and birth
(implanting more embryos and rejecting patients and/or surrogates they feel will
not be able to produce, which would negatively affect their success numbers),
and the use of testimonials, referrals, marketing materials, websites, and word-
of-mouth advertising.

Interpersonal trust between surrogates and IPs is more nebulous and difficult
to create through marketing strategies. As other scholars have shown, "trust
eases cooperation," is a "lubricant" for social interactions (Levine 2013, 35), and
"is often considered the 'glue' that holds society together" (van den Bos et al.
2011, 243; see also Fukuyama 1995 and 1999). Trust in interpersonal relations—
sometimes called "relation-specific trust" (as compared to a "general trust" or
"public trust" in systems, government, or organizations) is "generally defined as
a belief by a person in the integrity of another individual" (Larzelere and Huston
1980, 595; see also van den Bos et al. 2011). Katinka Bijlsma-Frankema and Ana
Cristina Costa have found a general consensus among scholars that "positive
expectations and the willingness to become vulnerable are critical elements to

define trust" (2005, 261). How do surrogates and IPs come to trust each other, to see each other as possessing integrity, to expect positive outcomes from their interactions with each other, and to be willing to engage in a relationship so fraught with risk and vulnerability? Frankly, some do not. Interpersonal trust between surrogates and IPs is not necessary for surrogacy to occur. Think of the Indian example at the beginning of this chapter. Indian surrogates and their foreign IPs do not establish interpersonal trust with one another—in most circumstances, they do not even know each other, having no or very limited interaction with one another. Rather, in India each party cooperates because of self-interest (IPs want babies, and surrogates want money). As Francis Fukuyama argues, "trust is not necessary for cooperation," but self-interest combined with a system of contracts "can compensate for an absence of trust and allow strangers jointly to create an organization that will work for a common purpose" (1995, 26). Indian surrogates and their IPs establish relationships with agencies, clinics, and caretakers—but generally not with each other—and operate within the regulations of the industry. In similar ways, if surrogates and IPs in the United States do not trust each other, the rules of the industry formalized through the contract take on an added level of importance in ensuring that both parties cooperate with each other. Fukuyama notes the importance of "formal rules and regulations, which have to be negotiated, agreed to, litigated, and enforced, sometimes by coercive means," when people do not have interpersonal trust (ibid., 27).

Surrogates and IPs can have a more formalized business arrangement with little interaction in the United States if they so desire. In the early years of surrogacy in the United States, closed programs—in which the identities of surrogates and IPs were not disclosed to each other—allowed for such arrangements (Ragone 1994). Today, the parties might have to work outside of an agency (most of which require interaction between surrogates and IPs) and have an independent arrangement. The surrogates and IPs in my study all expressed an interest in interacting with each other. For surrogates, it is those relationships that "make" surrogacy. Some of the IPs I have spoken with also found those relationships important and fulfilling. For others, their desire for interaction can be partially explained by the fact that unlike India, where formal regulations and disparities in power and money bind surrogates to their agreements, in the United States contracts alone are not enough to mitigate all of the risks and ensure that all parties abide by their agreements and behave in ways conducive to smooth interpersonal relations. Rather, interaction that facilitates trust (or a feeling of trust) is needed. It is the "near-constant presence of risk that creates the need for trust" (Levine 2013, 36).

The literature on trust identifies several important ways that interpersonal trust is established. Trust in relationships of familiarity is sometimes called "characteristic similarity" or "character-based trust" (Bijlsma-Frankema and Costa 2005, 261; see also Levin 2013). Those who come from similar life situations, social spheres, or institutions to our own may seem more trustworthy than others because of that similarity, even if we do not know them personally. So, for example, Americans abroad may strike up an instant friendship and display a level of trust in each other based purely on their shared nationality. For the most part, surrogates and IPs let me know that they did not come from the same social circles or life circumstances. But, as noted above, surrogates attempt to reach a trusting relationship by making the most of hobbies or interests that they share with IPs. The fact that surrogates and IPs have been vetted and selected by agencies helps as well. The rituals of the psychological, criminal, and medical screenings in particular assure both IPs and surrogates that the other party has been scrutinized and should be considered trustworthy.

Judith Levine's (2013) recent study on low-income mothers and their experiences in the welfare system highlights another route to trust. Repeated interactions over time with others (at work, in social institutions, or with friends and family) can promote (or inhibit) trust, Levine argues. This is called "process-based trust" (Bijlsma-Frankema and Costa 2005, 261). Unlike other types of relationships that build (or destroy) trust over time, however, commercial surrogates and IPs commit to each other (and to surrogacy) after having known each other for a relatively brief period. In many cases, the amount of interaction they have had with each other is minimal (a phone call, some e-mails, relatively brief meetings) before they sign contracts. They are essentially strangers to each other at the beginning of a new journey, yet they are asked to commit to the other party in a fairly risky venture.

Though surrogates and IPs make a leap of faith at the beginning, the interactions they have with each other over time promote or impede trust, which directly affects their experiences with surrogacy. Many surrogates and IPs told me that interpersonal trust is vital for positive experiences. Surrogates in particular work hard to appear trustworthy. One important way they do so is by attempting to communicate pure motives for becoming surrogates. This can be seen in the language they use when talking about the children created via surrogacy and their relationships to them. Surrogates generally find it repugnant for women to renege on their agreements. They emphasized to me that they did not engage in surrogacy because they desired more children. Surrogates are women who generally achieve pregnancy easily and give birth without issue. Surrogates do not need surrogacy to have another child. "If they wanted another baby," people often told me, surrogates "would just have one. They don't need to go through all of this to have a baby." Instead, surrogates expressed a commitment to the field of surrogacy in general and a deep individualized commitment to their IPs. This was true even when their IPs disappointed them or when they were having serious disagreements. According to my interviews, surrogates come to care—in some cases, quite deeply—for their IPs and to sympathize with their struggles to achieve a live birth. Treena Winmer captured this sentiment when she talked to me about how her two surrogacy pregnancies (both with twins) differed from her pregnancies with her own two children: "You do everything you can to make sure it's right, even more so than you would if it were your own. Because you know how much they have to trust you to do it." She went on:

I can't just say, "Well, these [babies] aren't mine. I'm going to do what I want anyway because I'm not going to be stuck with them." You don't do that. It's the same thing as watching [someone else's] child in your house. You take better care of that child because you want them to go home perfect. The same thing. It's the same goal. . . . Your goal at the end of the nine months is to get that healthy happy child that you've worked nine months to give . . . [and because of that] you go above and beyond. You feel that on a daily basis, which is a good thing. Keeps you grounded and reminds you, don't drink that Coke you want. Don't eat that third bowl of ice cream you want! (laughing)

Many surrogates shared similar comments with me about the care they take with their surrogacy pregnancies: watching what they eat, being careful of secondhand smoke, not lifting heavy items, stopping outside work earlier in the pregnancy, checking with their obstetricians regarding any issues of concern, and just generally being more cautious than usual—and even more cautious than they were during their pregnancies with their own children. They spoke of the "precious cargo" they carried and the responsibility of ensuring the safe arrival of their surro-babies both as a duty and a privilege.

Surrogates were emphatic that they did not want their surro-babies to be their own. Part of their work as surrogates involves communicating this idea to their IPs and to others who may be skeptical about surrogacy. Surrogates were well aware that IPs and others witnessing the surrogacy had concerns about their absconding with the babies. They worked to calm those fears by using specific language when talking about the pregnancy to others to signal their emotional distance from the babies. From the beginning of their journeys, the surro-babies were their IPs', not their own, they told me. They would use that language with their IPs, referring to their surro-babies as the IPs'. Jessica Klein captured this sentiment well:

I just went into this knowing, "This is not my baby. It's [my IPs] Gia and Charles's baby." Or this time it's [my new IPs] Trista and Oscar's baby. And I care about them, and I'm going to eat right and I'm going to sleep and do what I need to do, take my vitamins—but I have a love for them but kind of like [for] my nephews. And a lot of people don't understand that. "How can you not want them?" Well, I don't want them. I want them to go home and I want to go visit them, but I don't want them because they're not mine.

Like Jessica, many surrogates spoke of the love they have for their surro-babies as being similar to their love for their nieces or nephews, or for the children of their good friends. They insisted that their surro-babies are not their children; this was made easier for Jessica, who was pregnant on her second journey, as it was for most of the women in my study, by the fact that she did not contribute her own egg to the creation of the baby. Jessica stated: "I think that's an easier thing for a gestational surrogate versus traditional because if that was my egg right here, that would be so hard for me. I would be crying right now, knowing I have to give this baby away one day. But as my friend Shannon said, 'At delivery you're just giving their babies back to them. You just grew them, now you're giving them back.'" The idea of "giving their babies back," that their true parents are the IPs, regardless of the role that the surrogate played in giving them life, is an important one in contemporary surrogacy. Like Jessica, most surrogates clearly distinguish between their own genetic children and the children of their IPs, whom they simply gestate and bear—with a good deal of care and trust.

The care that surrogates take with their pregnancies is not simply because they are carrying someone else's child; it is also because of the trust placed in them coupled with the heightened importance of carrying a baby for someone who has experienced infertility. As discussed in chapter 2, most IPs have experienced infertility and heartbreak in attempting to achieve a live birth, and surrogates are sensitive to this. Rosalyn Whelan spoke about the empathy surrogates need to have for the long battle waged by their IPs to have a child and the need for surrogates to allow themselves to feel their IPs' pain:

> It's a very long road to get to where they are, and you have to be completely understanding of so many different situations because you don't know what they've been through. And so you aren't infertile, but you have to be in a way, it's like you immerse yourself in the world of infertility. So if you don't understand it, you'll never really have a good and successful match because if you don't empathize with them, you're not ever really going to click. Like you really do have to understand where they're coming from and get down on their level and really feel what they're feeling. Otherwise it's just kind of like, why would you do it? If you can't understand their heart and the wanting, it is kind of hard to imagine going through all the pain and all the procedures and stuff.

Rosalyn speaks of empathy as an important way of bonding the surrogate both to her individual IPs and to the process of surrogacy. Note that Rosalyn asks why would you do surrogacy, if you cannot "really feel" what the IPs are feeling in terms of their infertility struggles and their deep desires for a child? Disregarding the monetary exchange, Rosalyn is identifying empathy and the surrogate-IP relationship as a motivator for women to engage in surrogacy. Working together and sharing the highs and lows of attempting to achieve and sustain a pregnancy drew many surrogates and IPs closer together. Surrogates' empathy for their IPs encouraged new conceptualizations of their fertility invincibility and allowed them a deeper understanding of the pain of infertility.

The challenge, of course, is that most surrogates have no prior experience with infertility. This was the case for all of my participants except one. Working with their IPs was their first venture into the land of infertility, and it was difficult. Surrogates saw themselves as possessing intrinsic, special skills related to pregnancy and birth. They had never experienced any difficulties getting pregnant themselves, and most had enjoyed uneventful deliveries of their own children. They understood themselves to be good at pregnancy and were proud of their skills. As gestational surrogates, however, they attempt to achieve pregnancy using the gametes of their IPs, who have experienced infertility. For the first time in their lives, they experience the frustration that comes with trying to conceive and having negative pregnancy tests.

Surrogates come to gestational surrogacy with the expectation that their own fertility would transfer to their IPs, and some are shocked when this does not happen. Angela Cross shared with me her feelings about dealing with the negativity that IPs develop after repeated disappointments. "That was so hard for me," Angela said, "because I'm not a negative person at all. I try to see the positive in every situation." Angela approached the surrogacy with the belief that "oh no, this is going to work. It will be fine." But her IPs did not believe her. They could not trust in the process after all of the disappointments they had faced. Angela went on: "I mean, they were talking about it would be more likely for us to walk on the moon than to have a baby. They were just so convinced that it wasn't in their cards. And I think when it finally did happen they were super excited, but then [they thought], 'Wait a minute. This can't be good. Something bad is going to happen.' Like, [they were] always waiting for the other shoe to drop." And, unfortunately, sometimes the other shoe does drop.

Surrogates experience failed transfers, chemical pregnancies, miscarriages, stillbirths, and fetal death—in many cases, for the first time in their lives. Women seemed to take these failed surrogacy attempts personally. The responsibility they assumed for their body's ability to achieve pregnancy coupled with the sympathy they felt for their IPs culminated for many in feelings of guilt when pregnancy and a live birth was not achieved. This sentiment was captured by Josephine Maselli when she shared with me how she felt during her current surrogacy journey, her second with the same couple for whom she had borne a singleton. After three unsuccessful embryo transfers, Josephine was at an emotional low point:

It's been really hard for me that it's not working. I keep wondering if there is something wrong with me. They've done all the tests on me. There is nothing left to do. But still it's like—like when they put four embryos in and I didn't get pregnant, it was like, they trusted me with four little lives and it was so hard that I lost them—like, I felt like I lost them. So that's one thing. And some women think, "Oh I got pregnant so easily with my own, you know, I'll get pregnant." But they have to remember that there's a lot more to it. It's not just cut and dry. . . . I think emotionally that . . . the hardest part is when it hasn't worked. I mean it worked [on the first journey] like the way it was supposed to. That was easy. Now that it's not, it is emotionally very hard.

Josephine had become quite close to her IPs and was feeling their disappointment at each negative pregnancy test acutely. Like the other women in my study, she initially saw herself as the antidote to her IPs' continual pain. When she was unable to overcome their infertility, she took it quite personally.

Though surrogates told me that they were shocked by negative pregnancy tests, chemical pregnancies, and miscarriages, most IPs were not. Many IPs had actually come to expect failure. They were disappointed, of course, but not surprised. Sometimes the IPs actually comforted the surrogates for their own lost pregnancies. But sometimes surrogates were devastated by what they interpreted as the almost blasé attitude of their IPs to a negative pregnancy test or a miscarriage. Those moments were particularly painful ones in the relationships between surrogates and IPs. This became clear during the time I spent with Amanda Wagner, a two-time surrogate who had just experienced a stillbirth due to HELLP syndrome (the name comes from its symptoms: hemolysis, or the breaking down of red blood cells; elevated liver enzymes; and low platelet count), a potentially life-threatening condition (for both infant and gestating woman) thought to be a form of severe preeclampsia, which necessitates the immediate delivery of the infant. While Amanda was grieving the loss of the pregnancy and death of the infant, she was also dealing with the physical repercussions of the medical emergency. And she felt as though her IPs had already moved on to considering the next step in their desire to have a child—and doing so on a Hawaiian vacation. This bothered Amanda, especially because ongoing medical issues meant that she had had to return to the hospital the evening before speaking to me. She said: "I was just so fed up last night. I was talking to my dad and I was just like, 'For me it hasn't ended. I'm still having problems.' But for my IPs it has. And I know they have their own problems, but they're already on their vacation. Which I didn't mind them going [on], don't get me wrong. Until last night [when I returned to the hospital]. I'm like, 'Well, why am I still dealing with this? They get to be out there in Hawaii.'"

Implicit in Amanda's complaints about her IPs' Hawaiian vacation was a class issue. Amanda understood that her IPs were grieving. They had been highly invested in the pregnancy, with the IM attending every medical appointment. Amanda couldn't quite understand, however, how her IPs could so quickly move onto Hawaii after the funeral of their daughter: "After they're done with [the funeral], it's completely done for them. And they can look forward to what they're going to do next to complete their family. But me, I'm still going to be dealing." In addition to the physical and emotional repercussions for Amanda, part of "dealing" with the loss of the pregnancy was financial. Amanda had bought a new vehicle when she had become a surrogate, banking on her compensation to pay the vehicle loan. As we sat talking the day after her release from the hospital, Amanda had an eye on the door, waiting for the mail, hoping a check from her IPs would arrive. There was a basic inequality in the picture: after the fetal death her IPs were on a tropical vacation while Amanda worried about her health and her finances.

Most IPs, like Amanda's, have long battled infertility. Surrogate professionals told me that this sometimes translates into an inability for IPs to trust the surrogacy process or their surrogate and to constantly being prepared for failure (for example, by refusing to participate in obstetrician visits or prepare a nursery for a child). This can result in what surrogates may interpret as keeping a cold distance or not having a "proper" response to failure. Some surrogates reported concerns because their IPs did not seem to be all that interested in the pregnancy or they appeared to be emotionally distant after a miscarriage. For example, Jessica Klein told me that when she was miscarrying her IPs' baby, "they were off at the lake with their friends . . . and it didn't bother them because they kind of distanced themselves, knowing that that was going to happen." Jessica realized that "they had been through it before, so it was no big deal." However, she admitted, "that was hard. That was definitely hard." Several surrogates reported similar behavior at the birth of surro-babies. Some IPs did not attend the birth or seem concerned (in the estimation of their surrogates) that they were not there to witness such an important event. Other surrogates reported that their IPs did not remain with their newly born children after birth but instead left the hospital to nap, shower, or relax at a hotel. The surrogates whose IPs behaved this way found it disturbing. April Palmer, for example, was upset when her IPs left after their son was taken to the neonatal intensive care unit (NICU) after birth. According to April, her IPs "went home to take a nap and to take a shower, [and] that was actually really hard for me." April went on:

> I still don't know why they did that. But I was shocked and surprised because I thought, "If it was my baby that I just gave birth to, you don't leave the hospital because they go into the ICU!" And I didn't understand how they could do that. So I did call our program psychologist about it because it upset me. Not to the point where I was in tears or anything. I was more confused. And when she said there were lots of different psychological reasons why they may have felt the need to disconnect at that moment . . . but for me I was just pretty shocked and surprised.

Distancing themselves from the pregnancy is one method IPs use to deal with the risks and emotional pain that may occur with surrogacy. Another strategy used by some IPs to deal with the inherent risks is attempting to retain some semblance of control over the pregnancy through the micromanagement

of surrogates. For some surrogates, control was a serious issue in their relationships with their IPs.

The women in my study spoke of several ways in which surrogates felt "micromanaged," as they put it, during the surrogacy process. For example, sometimes
there is a constant barrage of phone calls, e-mails, and texts from IPs during
which surrogates are questioned on the minutiae of their eating, sleeping, and
activities and on any indications they might be feeling of changes in the pregnancy. Rhonda Chapman, a one-time surrogate of twins, was careful to avoid
this type of micromanagement. She spoke with distain about arrangements in
which "the IM has called [the surrogate] every day and they're practically in for
a two-hour conversation every time, reciting what they had to eat, and they'd
better not be eating hotdogs because of the nitrites. I mean, all sorts of things."
None of my participants desired this type of intrusion into their daily lives, especially because they view it as an indicator of a lack of trust and of respect for the
skilled care they bring to surrogacy. Most, however, were sympathetic to IPs who
needed constant communication about the pregnancy. Allison Farro's statement
was typical of the compassion surrogates have for IPs: "I understand the couples
that are paranoid and calling all the time because they have no control over the
situation. They have left something this big in someone else's hands and they
don't have any control other than to be pains, to call constantly and assert some
sort of control over the doctor or what the surrogate is doing. I understand the
psychology behind it." Like Allison, most other women were patient with their
IPs. But sometimes they felt their IPs were "out of control," and they needed the
agency to step in and help manage the situation. This is another important role
many agencies take on: the management of interpersonal conflict between IPs
and surrogates.

This management was especially evident at other times when surrogates also
sometimes felt controlled: during the contract phase or when unexpected decisions needed to be made and they felt as though their IPs did not trust their
judgment. This was especially tricky when these were new health care decisions
regarding the pregnancy that had not been previously discussed or addressed
in the contract. Surrogates understand themselves to possess important skills
and knowledge about pregnancy and birth gained through their in-depth experience. They see themselves as experts of a sort, especially when comparing
themselves to IPs, many of whom have never achieved pregnancy. This arose
during my interview with Cindy Woltz, a five-time surrogate and mother of two
who worked as a surrogate for the decade from her early thirties to her early
forties. Cindy's attitude toward her controlling IM was: "Oh please. I did this
in my sleep. Don't try to tell *me* how to carry a pregnancy." Cindy and her IM
eventually had an altercation over the length of time Cindy should take a particular medication to deal with a pregnancy-related medical issue. The IM did
not believe that Cindy and her obstetrician were displaying proper concern over

her developing baby. Cindy described the interaction with her IM: "She stood in my living room and had the biggest tantrum ever seen. Because she wanted me to keep taking those injections even though the doctor said, 'No, she's not taking them. It's not necessary, as a matter of fact it's dangerous.' . . . Oh, it was so awful the way she said, 'You're going to kill my baby. Do you realize you're killing my baby?'"

Cindy and her IM had the same goal: a successful pregnancy and a live birth. However, the heightened investment, the deep concern, and the loss of control over the pregnancy seemed to push this IM to the edge. Surrogates are sympathetic to their IPs, but many in my study reacted strongly to the lack of respect they feel—given their own knowledge of pregnancy, birth, and understanding their own bodies—in such altercations. For example, Ashley Padilla, a twenty-five-year-old who had five children of her own and was on her second surrogacy journey, emphatically argued against the presumed expertise of IMs regarding pregnancy: "I don't need somebody to tell me how to be pregnant! This isn't my first rodeo! It sounds kind of harsh to say, but you see these IPs who are micromanaging the surrogate who has four kids and they've never had any. And it's like, 'What are you doing?!'"

Surrogate professionals warn IPs about micromanaging surrogates. Control issues can result in IPs not being matched with a surrogate or with surrogates cutting off contact with IPs or refusing to let them participate in obstetrician visits or the birth of their children. It can also lead to surrogates making more demands in terms of compensation or other stipulations in their contracts. For example, Treena Winmer's IM asked her if she would consider having her artificial nails removed because of the chemicals used. Though Treena had worn such nails "all [her] life," including during her pregnancies with her own two children and her first surrogacy pregnancy, she agreed. After all, she said to me, "they're not asking me to cut my hands off!" However, "on the flip side of that, I said [to my IM], 'I will do that, of course. If that's something you would do for yourself, I will do that. But if you're afraid of the chemicals, then would you give me a house cleaner? Because I clean my house every week." Treena described this as a "give-and-take situation: I take off my nails, we have a house cleaner." Treena explained this exchange as tit for tat. Others described similar interactions. Some IPs are conscious of this and warn others, as did Renee Tillman, an IM I interviewed, "as the intended parent, you don't want to be a control freak. You can't control everything. So you need to really have trust in the person, remember why you selected them, and give them—you trust them, so give them space, don't be all over them."

Experienced surrogates are cautious about agreeing to work with IPs who appear to have micromanagement tendencies. Deidre Richards has experience with this issue both as the owner of a small surrogacy agency and as a surrogate herself: "The biggest complaint that I hear from surrogates is how the parents are trying to micromanage everything." She told me about one couple who came to her agency as new IP clients and wanted their surrogate to eat organic food and use green cleaning products. Deidre conceded that those were "all great things, but the chances of finding a surrogate that's going to do that?! That's very difficult." She went on: "Going into a relationship with a couple that came with a list of demands like that would probably scare me away a little bit. Not that I'm going to do anything bad, but you want to make sure that you uphold the contract and uphold the intended parents' views of what they want . . . that's got to be a tremendous amount of pressure. And I think it would be very difficult to work with someone like that." On the flip side, quite a few surrogates commended their IPs on their lack of micromanagement tendencies. Deanna Meer, for example, was in awe of the trust her IPs placed in her: "My couple is very trusting. They don't ever ask what I'm eating. They don't ever ask what I'm doing." Deanna loved this aspect of her journey, especially as she had heard from other surrogates about the micromanagement and control issues they were experiencing. "You hear all these stories," she told me, "because we go to support group meetings every month with other surrogates in the program, and you hear some of these horror stories about 'Well, are you eating this? You need to do this.' Just really on top of them." In contrast, Deanna's IM said to her: "You have two kids. They're perfect! What are we worried about?" The "total trust" and "faith" they placed in Deanna, she told me, is "very humbling."

Like Deanna, some women formed relationships with their IPs in which they felt supported and trusted. Trust is essential for a smooth journey, and displays of lack of trust can be problematic. As Tara Akerman, an IM on her first journey, cautioned, "you have to trust the person that's doing it for you. You have to trust the surrogacy agency. You have to just open yourself up to that because there are no guarantees. Nobody is going to monitor someone's nicotine intake. Just things like that that you have a million questions about. Nobody is going to do that thing so you have to make sure that you're matched correctly. And then you have to trust." As Tara stated, "good matches" are essential for the functioning of surrogacy.

Others were disappointed by a lack of connection, support, and trust. However, some surrogates were sensitive about appearing too needy to their IPs and to others witnessing their relationship. Sherry Woods, a one-time surrogate, was critical of surrogates on this issue. "Some of them," she said to me, are surrogates "just because they crave the attention" or because "something is lacking in their lives, and they're doing this because it makes them feel needed and important." Sherry saw this translate into surrogates "complaining about how horrible their IPs are and that they don't pay any attention to them and blah, blah. . . . There is an underlying neediness with a lot of them." Sherry distanced herself from that kind of surrogate: "I've got my whole own life to live. I don't really need someone calling me constantly and checking up on me."

Surrogates let me know that they sometimes had difficulty knowing how to proceed in their relationships with their IPs. They wanted their IPs to be involved and enjoy the process, but they did not want constant surveillance. They wanted to be trusted to care properly for their gestating surro-babies, but they also wanted their IPs' attention. Sometimes it was challenging to strike the right balance, especially because the IP-surrogate relationship often changes during the course of a surrogacy journey. The period directly following the birth of the surro-baby is when this issue becomes most evident and has the potential to cause considerable problems for both surrogates and IPs.

POSTPARTUM

As is the case with many kinds of relationships, the surrogate-IP relationship often evolves over the course of months or years, since it can take that long to achieve a live birth. Most of the surrogates had frequent pregnancy-related interactions with their IPs during the journey—sometimes, as will be discussed in the following chapter, involving their families—and more limited contact following the birth. Often, postpartum contact is in the form of e-mails or pictures, which some agencies "require" IPs to send to surrogates at certain intervals following the birth.[5] In addition to family pictures and updates, some surrogates receive annual gifts on their birthdays or flowers on Mother's Day from their IPs.

Some matches evolve into deep friendships with frequent contact that continues after the surrogacy concludes. This was the case with Jessica Klein. She and her husband, Aaron, had become close friends with her first set of IPs, for whom she bore twins. From the beginning of their journey, Jessica told me, both she and her husband "knew we want to be friends with these people forever." They had frequent contact throughout the pregnancy with her IPs. Jessica's entire family, including her two young children, became close with the IP couple. In addition to pregnancy-related contacts, such as visits to the obstetrician, they spoke often on the phone, frequently visited each other's homes, and invited each other to family parties. Following the birth of the twins, the close relationship continued. When the twins were six months old, the IPs took Jessica and Aaron up on their offer to watch the children overnight. The Kleins babysat for a weekend while the IPs visited family members and spent time with their older child. From that point forward, the Kleins kept the twins for days at a time. Jessica also entrusted her own children to her IPs. They came to view each other as extended family. Several other surrogates in the study came to consider their IPs part of the family, sometimes using kinship terms with each other (with the surrogate usually being called aunt). They meet often with their IPs or plan visits yearly if they live some distance away. Laurel Molza, for example, said: "It's really cool to develop those relationships. I've made some great friends. I will have lifelong friendships with most of the parents."

This level of continued closeness, especially that similar to the kind forged by Laurel and Jessica and their IPs, was unusual in my sample. Most surrogates had more infrequent contacts with their IPs following birth, consisting of e-mails or annual holiday updates. Many understood the decrease in contact to be a natural progression of the relationship. And the naturalness of the relationship was a key. Though Tina Vargas, for example, would like to hear from her IPs more often, "at the same time, I still know where I stand as far as they're still thankful and they're still glad, but they're just going on with their life. And that's fine." This was a common sentiment among surrogates, especially those who had been on multiple journeys and is one that is advanced by agencies. April Palmer captured this idea.

> I didn't really have an expectation as far as relationship afterward. I felt then and feel now, in my third surrogacy, that it's really not about me, it's about them. So whatever works for them is fine with me. Obviously during the pregnancy you want them to be as involved as possible because you want them to have that experience, because you've had it with your kids and it's awesome. But afterward if they just wanted to send pictures once a year or not at all, that would be okay with me. I've really felt like whatever they have to do to be comfortable to move on in their lives with their family is fine with me. So I didn't really have any expectations. I have always thought that a relationship will either develop or not during the process. And if it does and you're really close with someone, then great, probably carry that on. And if it doesn't then you've still done something awesome, and they still know that. Just because they may not want to have a relationship with you, I'm sure that they think about you because you gave them their dream. So it's never been that big of a deal to me.

Problems arise, however, when surrogates feel as though they had been led to expect a certain level of contact with their IPs and that has not come to fruition. Tina Vargas has heard, "Oh yeah, we'll stay in touch. We'll stay in touch," from IPs, "and then the surrogate has the babies and that's it. They won't call. [The surrogate will] call and they won't get back in touch with them. And then [the surrogate and her family were] kind of like, 'We thought we were going to stay in touch. I thought I didn't do anything wrong.'" This is particularly painful because of the time, energy, and sacrifice surrogates feel they have made on behalf of their IPs (Berend 2012). Having framed their relationship as a love match, they now came to understand IPs' true feelings about their arrangement: it is a business transaction. As will be discussed in greater detail in the next chapter, this is particularly problematic when surrogates' children are involved.

Some surrogates reported a dramatic "change of roles" following birth. Whereas during the pregnancy, the surrogate was the center of attention and information, after the birth, she is no longer. Dawn Rudge shared with me how disorienting this was for her. "All of a sudden you go from having full control to having absolutely no control. You kind of switch roles. All of a sudden instead of being the one that gives all the information and is kind of the center of it all, you're the one on the outside waiting to get information." Most of the surrogates felt this way. Because of this, the time period immediately following birth was disorienting for them. This sometimes revealed itself in the issue of being able to hold the child, which some women report gives them a sense of closure. Erin Peters experienced this on one of her journeys when the IPs did not give her the opportunity to hold her surro-baby, something Erin regrets. During her most recent journey, she thought, "Well, I'd like to hold the baby. Do I wait for them to offer? Do I ask?"

> So here I am waiting, and then they didn't know if I wanted to hold the baby because they didn't know if I was going to have a hard time with the attachment issue. So they were waiting on me to say something! So finally, here we are, five minutes from me going home and I said, "Can I hold the baby?" And we both busted out laughing because we're like, "Well, we were waiting on you. And we were waiting on you." It was ridiculous! They would have let me hold the baby for the last two days if I wanted! Silly me. But it was fine because just getting to sit there and watch them was so cool. So my last experience was just neat. It was all that I could ask for really.

Erin's experience highlights the complexity of the postpartum period for both surrogates and IPs. Following birth, IPs are consumed with their new babies and the transition to parenthood. They have little time to care, physically or emotionally, for their surrogates. Nor are there clear cultural guidelines in terms of appropriate behavior. Some women took the transfer of the IPs' attention from themselves to the baby quite personally and felt used, but most had more pragmatic views of this transition period.

The period directly following birth is a time of heightened emotion and changing relations between surrogates and IPs. Surrogates are also experiencing the surges in hormones that follow birth, the effects of which can present themselves in sometimes dramatic displays of emotion. Surrogates are sensitive about this issue because they feel as though the general public has a misunderstanding of the emotions they may be feeling postpartum. Some women spoke of family members or friends who had deep concerns that the surrogate was mourning the loss of the surro-baby, when, they reported, they were actually dealing with hormones and missing the relationship with their IPs. Ann Beltran, a mother of four who had given birth on two surrogacy journeys when she was in her early thirties, spoke about this when discussing the feelings of loss she experienced postpartum: "It's not even with the baby! A lot of people try to make it be: 'Oh it's about the baby.' No. It's about the whole relationship that you have with the IPs. And I think at that point is where you're not talking to them all the time any more obviously. They're not calling you to see how you're doing . . . you're not that priority anymore." Ann went on to discuss how those feelings of loss can negatively affect some surrogates and encourage women to seek new IPs and engage in surrogacy multiple times: "I think a lot of surrogates have that kind of problem after [birth]. I can't tell you how many times I've heard that. And then they're upset with the IPs, instead of being happy with what they did and kind of just moving on from there. But they're still kind of, 'Oh, they don't call me. They don't send me cards and letters and pictures.' And yeah, that would be nice, but really! So I think that's why a lot of them will go and do it over and over again."

Confirming Ann's interpretation, other women used confessional or joking tones when telling me that they entered into repeat surrogacies because they enjoyed the attention from IPs and were seeking that type of supportive relationship again. Deanna Meer, for example, had originally intended to help only one family but then found herself drawn to becoming a repeat surrogate. "I never knew I'd do it more than once," she said, "even though it is addicting! You want to do it again and again and again." Others also likened surrogacy to an addiction, trying to find that "perfect journey," what Cindy Woltz described as "no bed rest, no bleeding, no drama of any kind, just quiet, calm," and lots of positive attention from IPs. Though some surrogates described their journeys in such terms, Cindy remarked: "I never got it, really. It was always, there was always this power struggle, either with me and the mom or with people not being engaged." Erin Peters, who was on her fourth journey when I met her, was chasing the perfect journey until her last. Though she finally did have what she saw as a final "great match," when I asked her what advice she would give to a women just starting out, she cautioned new surrogates "not to have the white picket fence thoughts. Like it's not going to be all sunshine and roses." Be realistic, she said: "Just because you think it's going to have this outcome and you're going to have this wonderful experience and you're going to be great friends and they're going to treat you well all the time and then you're going to get to see them, it may not happen." Several women were deeply disappointed and hurt when the promised continued contact with their IPs did not occur. They had originally thought they had found the "perfect match," but they found their relationship shifted once the IPs received their child. They thought they had fallen in love and made a deep life-long connection with their IPs, but they discovered that the IPs understood their relationship in more transitory, businesslike terms. This propelled some surrogates to match again with a new couple, in the hopes that their new journey would be the perfect one.

THE IMPORTANCE OF SMOOTH RELATIONS

As this chapter has explored, compatibility between surrogates and IPs—regarding ethical issues, interpersonal style, and desired amount of contact—is critical for the success of a surrogacy journey in the United States. Unlike the situation in India, where there is no expected contact between parties, in the United States there are high expectations that a relationship will be cultivated between surrogates and IPs. Surrogates are not housed in hostels in the United States with their movements monitored by clinics. Nor are they made vulnerable by economic desperation as they are in India. Rather, along with compensation, surrogates said that a personal investment in the practice of surrogacy and fulfilling interpersonal connections with their IPs are the aspects that draw them to surrogacy and encourage them to engage in repeat journeys. They enjoy surrogacy—they love it, they told me—because of the relationships they form with their IPs and because they can help their IPs have their much-desired children.

Surrogates, IPs, and surrogacy professionals are all invested in good interpersonal relations between surrogates and IPs, but for different reasons. Agencies attempt to make good matches to protect the integrity of the industry. Bad matches—for example, in which IPs and surrogates hold different views about ethical issues—could have destabilizing effects for individual surrogacy arrangements and for the industry as a whole. Because of the relative instability of the industry and lack of federal regulation, surrogates who renege on their agreements have the potential to draw considerable negative attention to the practice of surrogacy. Recall the effect the Baby M case, for example, had on the budding industry, as discussed in chapter 1. To protect their businesses, leaders in the industry now emphasize the importance of proper screening and match parties not only along the lines of similar perspectives on termination and selective reduction but on personality, relational style, and the stated amount of contact each party desires with the other. Bad matches are a lot of work for agencies, as they must scramble to keep the arrangements afloat. By ensuring good matches, the industry protects itself from negative publicity, overtime work, and possible legal entanglements. Andrea Tyson, the surrogate pressured into selective reduction, serves as a perfect example. Though she did offer to carry the twin pregnancy to term, despite any health challenges it might produce, and take legal responsibility for one of the babies, when her IPs decided they wanted to reduce to a singleton, Andrea did not flee but rather complied with their request. She had committed herself to her IPs and to helping them create the family they desired. She understood the surrogacy contract: the fetuses she was carrying belonged to her IPs, not to her. The exchanges she had with her IPs over the course of several years prior to the reduction had bonded her to them. That relationship was essential to enabling Andrea to follow through with the reduction even though she was personally devastated. As Andrea's experience demonstrates, smooth relations allow for greater cultural acceptance of the surrogacy industry. Andrea did not go public with the reduction, she did not file for parental rights, and she did not cause a fuss. Rather, she understood her place within the arrangement, and she kept her agreement. This was not a purely financial relationship. If it was, perhaps Andrea might have walked out. Instead, her emotional relationship with her IPs and her understanding of the surro-babies as her IPs' allowed her to uphold her contract. Though her case is dramatic, it represents the centrality of the surrogate-IP relationship to surrogacy in the United States.

IPs desire good matches and smooth interpersonal relations with surrogates not because they want to protect the industry, but because they want their babies in the end. They want to trust in the process, in the agency, and most importantly, in their surrogate to properly care for their child and hand him or her over after birth. Therefore, IPs evaluate the character of potential surrogates (and pay their agencies to do so as well) while in the matching process. Interpersonal interactions with surrogates allow IPs to witness the care women take during pregnancy. If IPs so desire, a good match also allows them to experience the pregnancy by proxy. They can attend doctor's visits, feel the baby kick (albeit from the outside), watch the growing bump, and hear about any changes, including their child's prebirth behavior. Some IPs cultivate deep and abiding friendships with their surrogates and enjoy their time together. However, the primary goal for IPs in this exchange is not to have a pleasant experience or to make good friends. An enjoyable pregnancy is not the goal: the goal is to receive a live baby. Smooth interpersonal relations are obviously not the only key to ensuring that outcome, but they do help.

Surrogates also want their IPs to achieve their goals of live children. However, surrogates desire good matches because they want to enjoy the pregnancy process with deserving, appreciative IPs. Many surrogates told me that they hungered for ideal journeys, which largely translate into close, authentic relationships between themselves and their IPs. All want to see the fruit of their labor, which is not the baby per se but the effect of the baby on their IPs. They want to witness the making of parents and recognize their important role in that process. This can be seen in the importance that surrogates place in the moment of transfer, the moment they hand over newborns to their IPs. Most women identified that specific moment as the reason they engage in surrogacy.[6] During my interviews with them, many women showed me a photograph of that moment or described it to me in depth and said, "This is why I am a surrogate." It is the relationship they have with their IPs and the fact that they are able to give these people who become special to them their much-desired children that women find so personally fulfilling. It is the positive, caring relationships with IPs; the care and attention surrogates receive; and the intrinsic value women place on their role as surrogates that give meaning to surrogacy for surrogates.

Fulfilling, compatible relationships between surrogates and IPs enable surrogacy to function in the United States. The Indian market model would not be culturally palatable in the United States. Rather, the market function of surrogacy needs to be appropriately obscured for these arrangements to be made in this country. This is made possible through the friendships and companionable relations that form between surrogates and IPs. Friends helping friends achieve their dreams is a far less stigmatizing activity than the industrial-like surrogacy hostels in India in which typically no relationship is cultivated between the gestating woman and the receiving parents, with the only link between them an exchange of cash for the baby. Surrogacy in the United States is framed by the industry and the community as a caring partnership in which "dreams come true," not as a baby factory in which economic exchange occurs. The relationships between IPs and surrogates function to bind surrogates to their agreements, giving IPs some peace of mind that their arrangements will not be violated, and to give both IPs and surrogates distance from the economic exchange in which they are engaged.

CONCLUSION

In a recent post on SMO, a surrogate counseled women just entering into surrogacy arrangements: "My advice is that you need to absolutely love your IPs. If you don't have an amazing connection with them, then it will be extremely, extremely difficult. Even with the awesome IPs I have, I still wonder sometimes if I was crazy when I decided to do this. But then I remember why I'm doing it for them specifically, and the anxiety goes away. This is not just a business contract. This is you deciding who should be a parent. That's a big responsibility, so you must love them." It is the love for her IPs that makes surrogacy more than "just a business contract" for this SMO poster and the women in my study. This function of the surrogate-IP relationship—the way it obscures the market function of surrogacy—is most evident when relations sour and the market comes to the forefront. Surrogates who experienced painful exchanges, lack of connection, or rocky relations with their IPs reported less satisfaction with the overall experience, explaining that they sometimes felt "used" and like a "paid worker." These problems are most acute when surrogates feel as though they are not given proper respect: when they are not trusted to behave with their surro-babies' best interests in mind, when they are micromanaged, and when their skills and knowledge do not seem to be appreciated. In these situations, surrogates report feeling like paid, unskilled help, rather than respected members of the baby-making team.

These are emotional and sometimes painful situations. Surrogates desire respect for their skills and the knowledge they bring to surrogacy. In this way, surrogates are similar to occupational communities, especially those in the process of professionalizing. Though surrogates do not talk about themselves as an occupational collective—in fact, they avoid linking themselves to each other as workers—they do think of themselves as a group, and they want that group to be respected. This can be seen in the comments of Laurel Molza when she argued that IPs "need to trust [surrogates'] instincts as well, that we know what we're doing. I know there's a few odd [surrogates] out there but for the most part we know our place, and maybe that's what it does come down to, part of the business arrangement." Trust—evidenced through respect and pleasant relations—Laurel argues, is part of the market exchange.

Feelings of respect and appreciation derive from the interactions surrogates have with others in the surrogacy world, especially their IPs. When problems arise in their relationships with their IPs, surrogates seek solace in several ways. The first is from their fellow surrogates. Surrogates have an occupationally based community in which they gain knowledge, share advice, seek solace, and celebrate the joys of their journeys. This community has its own language (for example, "ttc" for trying to conceive, "the 2ww" for the two-week wait, "surro-baby," and "IPs") and norms—in other words, its own culture—which is facilitated through online interactions, face-to-face meetings, and agency support group meetings. New surrogates are socialized via this community. Though surrogates are resistant to conceptualizing themselves as an occupational group, they do turn to the community of other surrogates for advice, understanding, and socialization and they think of themselves as a group and feel that they should be respected for their skills and knowledge.

The second way surrogates deal with difficult relations with their IPS is in remembering their original goals of helping someone achieve parenthood. As noted above in this chapter, at the beginning of most surrogacy journeys, IPs and surrogates are strangers to one another. Surrogates want the experience of attempting to help someone—not any person in particular—achieve parenthood. Some revert back to that anonymity, like Cindy Woltz, who experienced a sense of disconnection and uncomfortable exchanges with her IPs. After five surrogacies, Cindy came to the conclusion that "people are just people. And [IPs] disappoint us as much as we [surrogates] disappoint them. And my goals were met in the end. I helped four families have six babies. So how can you be disappointed in any of that? I mean, even all the horrible stuff that happened—we're all just people. And I have contact with all of them still. And I think for the most part they all appreciate what we did."

Other surrogates also spoke of disappointment as they reflected on their surrogacy experiences. Though there were women who told me that their journeys were "perfect," most experienced some disappointment, whether because of the behavior of IPs, sadness about a lack of continuing contact or connections, or feelings of distress or inadequacy over a failed journey. Part of surrogate work, then, involves the suppression or reframing of feelings and emotion—what Arlie Hochschild calls "emotional labor." Emotional labor "requires one to induce or suppress feeling in order to sustain the outward countenance that produces the proper state of mind in others" (1983, 7). Many surrogates let me know that they hid or attempted to hide their feelings of sadness or disappointment from their IPs because of the negative impact they might have on the journey.

Having worked in surrogacy for several decades, first as a surrogate and later as a surrogacy coordinator, Cindy understood the fallacy of the "perfect journey." "So just go into it and don't have any grandiose expectations," she advised, "because [otherwise] you'll be sorely disappointed." Rather, she counseled new surrogates to enter into surrogacy "for the joy of doing something for somebody, not that you're going to have this perfect pregnancy." Like other experienced surrogates, Cindy attempted to prevent newer surrogates from feeling disappointed by encouraging them to think about their work in a more self-protective way.

The "joy of doing something for somebody" is not the only way surrogates sought solace for unpleasant relations with their IPs and feelings of lack of respect for the work they do. As will be explored in depth in the following chapters, surrogates also take comfort in the fact that they are compensated and that they will have something to show for "all of the difficulties" their IPs "put them through." This is precisely why some agencies do not allow their surrogates to engage in surrogacy without compensation. The concluding chapter will show that agencies understand the symbolic importance of the monetary exchange in these complicated journeys.

As demonstrated in this chapter, satisfactory, fulfilling relationships between IPs and surrogates function to obscure surrogacy as work and the fact that money is being exchanged. Surrogacy is framed as a win-win situation in the United States, just as it is in India. However, in the United States, it is close, authentic relationships and positive experiences that are the goal of many surrogates as they seek perfect journeys with their perfect IPs. In an ironic twist, however, problematic relationships between surrogates and IPs, which make surrogates feel less like friends and more like paid unskilled workers, make the monetary exchange essential for surrogacy to function smoothly.

CHAPTER 5

Working from Home

SURROGATES AND THEIR FAMILIES

On a hot July day several years ago, I sat with Louis Vargas in his double-wide trailer in central Texas. The trailer was dim and invitingly cool, and Louis and his wife, Tina, who had been a surrogate twice (and was contemplating a third journey), were gracious hosts. It was my second trip to the Vargas home. Earlier, I had interviewed Tina about her birthing twins for two different couples. This time I was here to talk with Louis about his own experiences. I was interested in learning from surrogates' family members about how they experienced surrogacy and how they understood it to shape their own day-to-day lives. How did Louis feel about his wife carrying a pregnancy and birthing for another couple? What did Tina's four children think about their mother's pregnancies? Were Tina's family members involved in surrogacy, and how did they understand their experiences? These were some of the questions I pondered as I visited with Louis.

Through my interviews with surrogates I came to understand that including the perspective of surrogates' family members in my study was important. If I was going to understand contemporary surrogacy in the United States, surrogates told me, I would need to understand the role their families played. Most women were insistent that surrogacy work would not be possible without the support of a close ally—most often a husband or romantic partner. The temporal and emotional demands of surrogacy were too intense, I was told, without someone else to lean on. For example, Tina said that because surrogacy requires "a lot of time," she would not be able to be a surrogate without the help of her husband. "Like I've got to go to the doctor today," she explained. "I have to go do this or that, and that leaves him [responsible]." Some women also need assistance due to the physical demands of becoming pregnant through in vitro fertilization (IVF). This was the case with Tina. "The first three months," she told me, "because of all the hormone stuff, I'm on the couch. I can't move.

I can't do anything. So you have to have that family support that says, 'Okay, I will step in and cover your place.' You have to really have that." Surrogates rely on family members to both assist them with their surrogacy work and to pick up the slack at home due to the amount of time they spend away from their families for various doctor's appointments, support group meetings, social get-togethers, and visits with their intended parents (IPs). This chapter examines how those changes brought on by surrogacy work shape family life for surrogates, their husbands, and their children; what those experiences mean to the people involved; and what the experiences tell us about reproductive work and the contemporary family.

So I sat with Louis and sipped sweet tea as he recounted his family's two surrogacy journeys. My interview with Louis was one of my first with a surrogate's significant other, and it laid the groundwork for my subsequent thirteen interviews with husbands and other close family members. Through talking with surrogates' family members, I came to understand what a significant role surrogacy can play in their day-to-day lives and, for some, the important place surrogacy came to occupy in their own identities. Louis was very clear with me, for example, that surrogacy was something that he and his wife accomplished together. It was not "her journey" but "our journey"; not "her IPs" but "our couple." There was a lot of "we" talk in Louis's interview—"we decided this," "we chose that," and "we were happy." A good example of this was when Louis was sharing with me the criteria he and Tina used to choose "their first couple." Louis told me that they wanted an IP couple who had a true medical necessity for surrogacy:

> We weren't going to carry for somebody just because they didn't want to become pregnant. Some of the Hollywood people, where they don't have the time to become pregnant. So that was one of the things—we were not going to carry for somebody like that. We wanted some medical reason as to why you couldn't carry. We were definitely of the opinion that if your life is too busy for you to become pregnant—if you're capable of becoming pregnant—then your life is too busy to have a kid. [He laughed.] And again for our coping needs, we weren't going to go that route.

Notice that Louis refers to himself and Tina as jointly carrying the pregnancy ("we were not going to carry for somebody"). Louis even referred to himself as a "surrogate father." This was interesting because in the world of surrogacy the phrase "surrogate father" is devoid of meaning. Even in the larger world of assisted reproduction the term is not used. Men are fathers (biological and/or social) or they are sperm donors, but they are usually not referred to as surrogates. In popular speech the term "surrogate father" is most often used to denote a man who acts like a father toward someone. Louis, however, viewed himself in a complementary role: his wife was a surrogate mother, so he was a surrogate father. Though Louis was the only husband in my sample to refer

to himself that way, other men had a similar orientation to engaging in surrogacy along with their wives. They spoke of the decision making involved in
surrogacy and the subsequent pregnancy and birth as a collaboration—a joint
venture in which husbands and wives were both active participants. Though all
acknowledged that the main burden of surrogacy rested on surrogates' shoul-
ders, virtually all of the participants in my study mentioned the important role
that the surrogate's family, particularly her husband, plays in the surrogacy
experience.

Different players in the surrogacy industry appreciate men like Louis who are
engaged in the process and supportive of their surrogate wives. For example, the
American Society for Reproductive Medicine recommends that the surrogate
"should have a stable family environment with adequate support to help her
cope with the added stress of pregnancy" (2012a, 1304). Agencies follow these
recommendations, with many declaring that they prefer to work with women
who have "supportive home lives," signaling to potential surrogates a preference
for those in stable, monogamous relationships.

This preference can be seen in the demographics of my sample. Twenty-seven
of the thirty-one women in my study were in heterosexual romantic relationships. Twenty-six were married; one was cohabitating with a boyfriend. It is
difficult to determine if the marital status of my sample is representative of surrogates in the United States as a whole. As discussed above, no national data is
kept on surrogate demographics. The agencies with whose staff I spoke, however,
indicated that the majority of their surrogates were in heterosexual marriages.
Time spent in the field and in the world of surrogacy via surrogacy support
websites, blogs, and ongoing contact with surrogates taught me that although
there is variation in the sexual orientation and marital status of surrogates, the
public face of surrogates is one of heterosexual married women. This is a marketing technique, aligning surrogacy with notions of the "traditional family" by
attempting to mitigate what could be viewed as the transgressive nature of these
arrangements.

The presence of a legal spouse is not required for a woman to become a surrogate. There are single women without romantic partners who act as surrogates,
including four in my sample. Such women are accepted by many agencies as long
as they have what agencies characterize as a "supportive home environment." A
spouse who is unsupportive is much more problematic than no spouse at all,
as an unsupportive spouse could seek legal rights to any child his or her wife
bears. Some surrogacy professionals also expressed the belief that an unsupportive spouse could cause stress on the surrogate, which they viewed as having
the potential to negatively affect pregnancy. Some agencies refuse to work with
women who are in the middle of divorcing, especially if the separation is not
amicable. Women separating from their spouses have reported online that they

experience difficulty being accepted as surrogates by agencies due to potential problems arising with their soon-to-be ex-spouses.

While not all of my participants were married, all of them were mothers. Agencies and many reproductive endocrinologists (REs) require women to have given birth and to be raising or having raised at least one biological child. Surrogates' children are, therefore, necessary in surrogacy arrangements.[1]

As discussed above, surrogacy professionals identify two important reasons why surrogates are required to be mothers. First, surrogacy professionals want to ensure that women are capable of achieving and sustaining a pregnancy and giving birth. All parties involved in surrogacy—agencies, REs, and especially IPs—desire success. A live birth is the goal of IPs; and along with any altruistic impulses professionals might have toward IPs, live births are simply good business for agencies and REs. Therefore, time, energy, and especially money are not usually invested in uteruses that have not, as surrogacy professionals say, "been proven."

Having given birth to and raised (or be raising) a child is also required of surrogates because of the fears that exist about surrogates absconding with IPs' babies. Mothers, I was told, are assumed to better understand the potential challenges of gestating, birthing, and then parting with a child than women who have not experienced motherhood. Mothers are thought not only to possess specific mothering knowledge and therefore to better understand what they have agreed to in a surrogacy arrangement, but to be more sympathetic to IPs than non-mothers and therefore less likely to renege on their agreements.

The preference to use married mothers as surrogates has implications for both the structure and experience of surrogacy in the United States. Within the market, surrogates are not viewed only as independent workers but also as part of a familial unit—and that unit, especially its stability and likability, is a specific marketing tool used to entice clients and reassure practitioners. The surrogate family is also an entity that absorbs the labor of surrogacy. As I argue in this chapter, surrogacy becomes family work, not only because surrogates are working to, as surrogacy parlance puts it, "create a family" but also because their own families engage in labor related to surrogacy. This family work is reminiscent of the ways children assist with family-run businesses (L. Park 2005) or home-based work (Heck et al. 1995). As I will show in this chapter, surrogates' husbands and children participate in and are affected by various aspects of surrogacy. In this chapter I ask: How do surrogates feel about the impact their surrogacy work has on their families? And how do they negotiate the work-family conflict inherent in the time demands of surrogacy? An exploration of those experiences reveals that the involvement of surrogates' family members operates to reframe surrogacy as family sacrifice, rather than paid employment, thus helping to obscure surrogacy as work.

Permission—or, Who Am I to Stop Her?

My interviews with surrogates, their spouses, and other family members reveal that the decision to pursue surrogacy is often a family affair. Though the original impulse to investigate surrogacy usually originates with the surrogates, most women reported that they wanted their husband's consent and that they would not have engaged in surrogacy without their husband's full support. For example, Laurel Molza told me, "If at any point [my husband] had said no [to surrogacy], then that's not anything we would have pursued." Treena Winmer's husband, Joel, similarly noted that his wife "told me that unless I was on board completely [with surrogacy] that she wouldn't have done it." In the same way, many of the women I interviewed spoke of the decision to pursue surrogacy, and their marriages more generally, as partnerships. Although several women articulated decidedly traditional patriarchal orientations to decision making and marriage, the majority gave the impression that they had more of a give-and-take with their husbands, with most of their big, potentially life-altering decisions made jointly. This partnership and close communication between surrogates and their husbands is aligned with dominant notions of contemporary marriage in which "spouses are expected to be confidants and the main source of emotional support" (Gerstel and Sarkisian 2006, 19). Josephine Maselli, a one-time surrogate who was attempting a sibling project with the same IP couple, expressed this view when she told me: "I'm the type of person that even if [my husband] says it's okay, if I can sense that he's not fully supportive, I won't do it. I have to have him completely supportive of the choices I'm making. So he's there right with me, cheering us on, hoping this works." Most married women in my study reported that their husbands' support was vital for both their decision to pursue surrogacy and their ability to navigate the experience successfully.

Many participants in my study reported that they brought the idea of becoming a surrogate to their husbands when they began to seriously consider it. Typically, their husbands had heard about surrogacy before but were not aware of the different kinds of arrangements (gestational and traditional) and assumed that any children produced would be genetically related to their wives. Quite a few of the husbands, though they eventually became supportive, were initially resistant to surrogacy—in particular, to the idea of their wives conceiving, gestating, and parting with a biologically related child. This was not the case for all surrogates. Some had husbands or partners who were aware of gestational surrogacy and supportive from the start. A few women realized they wanted to be surrogates earlier in life, even before they met their husbands, and had already discussed this life goal with the men they later married. Most women in my study, however, first brought the idea to their husbands after they had birthed what they understood to be their last child. Becoming supportive of their wives' participation in surrogacy was, therefore, a process for most of the husbands.

Husbands' resistance was problematic for women interested in becoming surrogates for several reasons. First, the structure of surrogacy arrangements via most agencies and REs in the United States requires the consent and involvement of the surrogate's spouse or romantic partner, if she has one. Due to concerns that the spouse of a gestating surrogate could seek legal rights to any infant she bears, most agencies require legally married partners to sign surrogacy contracts and agree to legally rescind any parental rights to surro-babies. Because of this, at the beginning of the screening process—before agencies agree to take on a woman as a surrogate—most agencies demand an initial declaration of support from spouses before moving ahead. Some agencies require this to occur in the context of a formal interview or a psychological session with a counselor or psychologist. In these meetings some agencies and REs require extensive discussions with spouses that communicate information about the structure, experience, and risks of surrogacy. Other agencies and REs only need short verbal confirmation with the partner over the phone or via e-mail, while others require only that the prospective surrogate communicate this information.

It took work for some of the married women in my study to get their husbands to support their decision to become surrogates. Cherise Armstrong, a three-time surrogate and director of a small surrogacy agency, noted that "it takes a special man" to agree to surrogacy for his wife and that "a lot of men don't understand it initially." This was the case with Sandra Foster, who had to convince her husband, Thomas, to even contemplate surrogacy. His initial reaction when she broached the topic of becoming a surrogate with him was, "Are you crazy!?!" Sandra immediately backed off and wrote a six- to seven-page "mini-thesis" explaining the medical and legal aspects of gestational surrogacy and addressing Thomas's main apprehensions. She left the document on Thomas's desk, allowing him to digest the information at his own pace. Sandra knew her husband well, and her strategy worked.

Other women used different approaches in attempting to convince their husbands to consider surrogacy. For example, Amber Castillo mentioned Isaiah, a little boy she and her husband knew whose parents had used IVF to become pregnant with him. Thinking about Isaiah helped Amber normalize the use of IVF and surrogacy to create children, and she used the example of Isaiah when talking with her husband as well: "I think for my husband, too, knowing that Isaiah was IVF, that's how I explained to him. 'It's the same way Isaiah was made in the lab.' It is what it is. I said, 'It's going to be their kid made in a lab. It's not going to be anything to do with us.' Because he had no idea." Some husbands did not want to know the specifics of the medical procedures involved; others needed all of this information before they decided whether or not they would support this new venture of their wives. Regardless of the methods used to address their husbands' concerns, there were common apprehensions about surrogacy held by family members.

The biggest roadblock women faced to gaining familial support for surrogacy was the misconception that gestational surrogates part with genetically related children. For example, Gillian Dorsey's husband, Nick, was completely against traditional surrogacy, stating: "Right from the beginning I said, 'This needs to be something that's entirely their child, not anything to do with us biologically.'" Note that Nick claims a biological position in the surrogacy equation ("us biologically"), as if his own genes were involved. This is intriguing, for even in traditional surrogacy—in which surrogates use their own eggs—surrogates' husbands' biological material is never intended to enter the surrogacy equation.

Nick's sentiments highlight a view prevalent among the husbands in my sample and supported in specific ways by the law: their wives' bodies, genes, and biological relatedness to others were not the women's alone but also the husbands' and part of a larger familial identity. This can be seen in ways that paternity and familial relatedness is assumed—socially and legally—for the spouse of a heterosexual gestating woman unless otherwise declared. And this is where the concerns about traditional surrogacy arise. Husbands displayed a protectiveness toward their familial borders, not wanting children biologically related to their nuclear family to exist in the world who were not a part—legally and socially—of their family. For example, Vanessa Moreno's husband, Steven, did not want the possibility of a child related to himself or his wife to exist in the world who was not legally and socially his own child. Surrogacy was a new concept to Steven when Vanessa originally explained it to him, when they were dating. "He had never heard about it or known anyone who did it or had a child through surrogacy," Vanessa shared. "So I had to explain the whole entire thing." Vanessa's mother had actually served as a traditional surrogate when Vanessa was a child. Now that she was married with children, traditional surrogacy was an arrangement that Steven was not comfortable with for his own wife and family. "[But] now with the science catching up with surrogacy," Vanessa noted, "[Steven] knew that it wasn't going to be our—my—child; whereas back then it was my mom's biological baby. So now it's not. So I think that helped—that was a little better for him to accept because it wasn't my child. I think if it was the same as it was back then that he wouldn't be as supportive." Note Vanessa's verbal slip here as well: initially structuring her sentence to state that the child "wasn't going to be our child," which she then corrected to "my child." In some important ways, surrogates as well as their husbands conceive of surrogacy as a familial venture.

Vanessa went on to note that Steven was particularly resistant to traditional surrogacy because she and her husband "didn't have a girl." Though Vanessa reported that she and Steven had completed their family and did not have plans to add more children (a position women are encouraged to reach before they become surrogates), Steven continued to long for a daughter. Vanessa thought it would have been particularly hard on Steven had she become pregnant with a biological daughter (through traditional surrogacy) for another couple. "Yeah, I think he would have had issues," Vanessa told me. That dilemma was solved due to the possibility of gestational surrogacy. "So we don't even have to think about [the child being biologically related to me], [we don't have to] talk about that. That's not an issue. So now that I think that it's not my baby, I have no biological ties, no blood ties, no nothing, I'm just a carrier, he's like, 'Wow. It's a great thing.' He's totally supportive."

Similarly, Amber Castillo's husband, Victor, was unaware of gestational surrogacy and initially quite resistant to the idea of his wife's serving as a surrogate because he believed children biologically related to his wife would be produced in the process. Unlike Steven, however, Victor did not articulate his concerns because of his own desire for more (sex-specific) children, but because he believed that any surrogate children born via his wife would be half-siblings to his own children. Victor couched his apprehension about traditional surrogacy in expressions of love for and protectiveness of his family:

> The thing is, we have kids, and I guess the number one thing about me is family. So like—maybe because I didn't have a whole lot of family growing up. So right now what means the most to me is my family. And genetically [my] kids would be related to that [surro-]child and that would be one of the things that I would not want. You know, hey, I feel like these kids have a right to know this kid at least because it's their half-brother or sister or whatever it would be. So yeah, I wouldn't be comfortable with that at all. And that would be the only reason [I wouldn't want her to be a surrogate]. It wouldn't be because I just want to be selfish or anything like that, I don't think. But we are a family, and if I had a kid out of wedlock or something like that, it would be a horrible thing. And then, naw, I wouldn't do it.

Note that Victor is resistant to traditional surrogacy because it would disturb his family in the same way he imagined an "out of wedlock" birth would do. This is telling. Several husbands reported concerns about traditional surrogacy because they understood it, like Victor, as analogous to an adulterous union between their wives and other men. Victor was clearly uncomfortable with his wife using her own eggs to conceive a surrogate pregnancy. This was true of all of the husbands with whom I spoke and, as I discussed in the previous chapter, with many of the surrogates themselves. In this resistance to traditional surrogacy, we can see how basic ideas about the family shape who's in and who's out of what is conceived of as a clearly bounded unit.

In the 1960s the anthropologist David Schneider (1968) wrote about the importance of blood in American concepts of kinship. Though family ties are also formed through the order of law (marriage and adoption), in the American kinship system it is the order of nature (biology, blood, and now genes) that is seen to be primary. A good example of this that Schneider provides is the ways in which family members can or cannot separate from one another—how one gets out of the family. Divorce is a great illustration: you can divorce your husband (a relationship established via a legal process), and he ceases to be related to you. He is no longer your husband; you and he are no longer family, legally or socially. You cannot, however, divorce your biological child—a relationship established via the order of nature, or shared biological matter. Actually, you can legally separate from your child and no longer retain parental rights. The child can be removed from your care and your parental rights rescinded, or the child can establish him- or herself as an emancipated minor through legal proceedings. In popular American concepts of the family, however, even mothers who are legally separated from their biologically related children retain a familial identity. They continue to be regarded as the mother—sometimes called the "real mother"—of even those children adopted by other people. As Schneider observed, the order of nature always trumps the order of law in folk understandings of the family. Under the rubric of these folk understandings, biological relatedness cannot be divorced away.

These ideas about blood, genetics, and relatedness run deep in the American psyche. They determine who is in the family, regardless of intent or even of how the legal system defines a familial unit. This is particularly evident in parent-child relationships that form outside of traditional biological routes and in the ways in which many of the participants in my study thought about traditional surrogacy. Victor, Steven, and the other husbands in my study, along with many of the surrogates themselves, viewed children conceived using a surrogate's egg as the surrogate's child, regardless of the intent of the IPs and the surrogate, or of legal decisions. In this paradigm, the social system of traditional surrogacy is seen to merely mask the true and natural relationship between mother and genetic child. This paradigm privileges the order of nature, positioning the genetic bond as natural and determining, governing the maternal bond, regard-less of the prebirth order filed with the court. Blood trumps intent.

What is interesting and takes us beyond Schneider here is the way the men in my study spoke of their own familial connection to the hypothetical child conceived of through traditional surrogacy. The men did not reject traditional surrogacy based only on their wives' shared biology with the hypothetical child, but also on their own—and their children's—familial connection to such a child. They argued against a disturbing of what they clearly treasured as the sacred bounded unit of their families. It was not the fact that surro-babies would be carried by their wives. The physical act of gestating and birthing a child for others did not disturb them; rather, the husbands in my study were resistant to the idea that their wives would share any genetic connection to those children. There are, of course, married women who do serve as traditional surrogates or as egg donors and help create genetic offspring for others. However, the husbands in my study only agreed to surrogacy because their wives were non-biologically related carriers and not genetic mothers to the surro-babies they birthed—and many of the surrogates in the study held similar views.

The distinction between traditional and gestational surrogacy shaped how women and their husbands imagined their connections to their surro-babies. Like Vanessa and Steven, other surrogates and their husbands claimed from the beginning of their journeys that their surro-babies "truly" were not their own because the surrogacies were gestational and not traditional arrangements. Those babies had a genetic and familial identity separate from theirs, they told me. This is not only true to them—as it is rooted in the order of nature and therefore, under folk understandings of kinship, undeniable—but, I would argue, it also performs the important function of creating distance between surrogates and their families, on the one hand, and the babies, on the other hand. Making this distinction allows surrogates to avoid any feelings of proprietary connection to the babies they carry. Those babies, surrogates told me, "truly" and "naturally" are the children of their IPs. Participants in my study would argue that they do not have to work to create distance, as they see it existing naturally. I would argue, however, that this position is in itself a distancing technique and a way to help guarantee that surrogates and their families do not form familial bonds with surro-babies.

It was this distance between surrogates and their surro-babies, enabled by the gestational nature of their arrangements, that allowed the husbands in my study to agree to surrogacy. The language my participants used to describe the process of men's agreeing to surrogacy was largely that of permission. For example, like the other husbands in my study, once Ashley Padilla's husband, Garry, understood that any children would not be genetically his wife's—and thus not related to his family—and he would be able to explain that to other people, he agreed to "allow" his wife to begin the surrogacy process. Ashley told me: "When I explained it to him, the whole genetics of the situation, [I said] that I wasn't a traditional surrogate, I'm not giving away [the baby], I'm just renting my uterus. Surrogates hate it when you say that, but that's what you're doing! I don't understand [why they object]! So he finally said, 'OK, that's fine.'" Many women, like Ashley, reported that their husbands "let" them become surrogates. While this language appears to be conservatively oriented and more in line with a benevolent paternalism in which husbands protect their wives (due to their wives' inability to do so themselves), interestingly, this "granting of permission" terminology was used both by the several couples in my study who seemed to hold more traditional views of marriage and those who leaned toward more egalitarian positions. When I asked Russell Peters, for example, how he felt when his wife, Erin, first approached him about her becoming a surrogate, he said: "I kind of let her, if she wants to do something—in my mind, even though we're married if she wants to do it, let her do it, as long as it's not detrimental to our marriage or our family. If she wants to do it, let her do it. So when she started exploring the idea, I was open to it. If it's something she felt that she wanted to do, then kind of like—who am I to say that she can't do it?" Russell's comments are intriguing. At one and the same time he is arguing that his wife has the right to engage in activities she sees fit ("who am I to say that she can't do it?") and that he grants her permission to act (he "lets" her do it). Victor Castillo had a similar reaction. Though his wife, Amber, reported that she needed his permission and support and would not engage in surrogacy without it, Victor told me that although he "was a little hesitant [about surrogacy] at first, Amber has been in the army and she's an American. And my whole philosophy—the way I thought was it's a free country, she can do what she wants to do." This quote reveals the way some husbands (and their wives) draw parallels between liberty and surrogacy. There was a tension, however, between this position and husbands' role in decisions about surrogacy. Most husbands played a part in their wives' decisions to pursue surrogacy; they "granted permission" and acted as sounding boards during the decision-making process. Rosalyn Whelan, for example, was able to become a surrogate only after she separated from her partner. "Once we officially separated," she told me, "then I kind of felt free, like I could do what I wanted. He would never have let me. So it was like my first step doing something that I just really wanted to do."

Husbands' willingness to support their wives in surrogacy was viewed as important for women's abilities to successfully complete the process of acting as a surrogate. Molly Hughes spoke of the significance of spousal support: "This is not an easy journey. And I remember someone posting on [the surrogacy support website] 'All about Surrogacy' that she was not married, she had a boyfriend and wanted to be a surrogate. And I just remember thinking, 'You cannot do this by yourself.' You can't. I couldn't. It's hard. It's draining. And the emotional support—and it's just something I couldn't do by myself." Using language similar to Molly's, surrogates commonly reported that the support of their husbands was essential and that the women would not engage in surrogacy unless their husbands consented. Most husbands also saw themselves as important to the decision-making process and surrogacy more generally. Rarer were husbands who presented themselves as peripheral to the decision of their wives to become a surrogate for the first time. Deidre Richards's husband, Mark, was one such husband.

When I asked Mark what he thought about surrogacy when his wife first seriously contemplated it, Mark positioned himself as "a neutral player." "I didn't want to push her into anything because there's certainly nothing in it for me to gain," he said. "But at the same time I didn't want to hold her back. So as she contemplated the process, as she looked into it, as it evolved, I guess my role was pretty neutral. I certainly told her I didn't have any problems with it. I thought it would be a great and wonderful thing to do. But I didn't encourage it, I didn't discourage it, I guess." There were other men in my study who saw themselves as outside players in the surrogacy journey (and still other men were presented in this way by their wives). These men trusted their wives, they let me know, to make appropriate decisions about what type of activities they wanted to engage in and to evaluate how it would affect their family life.

Most married women in my study spoke of feeling a similar level of support from their husbands to pursue their dream of becoming a surrogate. Deidre, for example, shared with me the fact that although Mark let her make up her own mind about whether to pursue surrogacy, he was "very supportive" once she decided to do so. Then she added: "I think he would be supportive of me if I told him I was going to fly to the moon. He's just very supportive of me anyway."

Regardless of the role husbands played in the decision to pursue surrogacy, their support and involvement in these arrangements was spoken of frequently by surrogates. Surrogacy was not seen as an individual activity engaged in by an autonomous person, but as something that could have profound impacts on families and relationships between surrogates and their spouses. Most husbands were therefore involved in the initial decision to pursue surrogacy, with most surrogates claiming that their husband's approval was necessary for them to begin the process of serving as a surrogate.

Surrogates in my study let me know that part of their husbands' decision making about surrogacy was an initial evaluation of the potential harm that could come to their wives and their families from the women's participation in this medical and social arrangement. Surrogates also let me know that husbands contemplated potential benefits.

SPOUSAL BENEFITS

Most husbands reported that they personally gained something from their wives' surrogacy experiences. Some men identified this as the compensation their wives were paid. While all of the surrogates in my study let me know that they did not engage in surrogacy primarily for the compensation they received, some of the husbands indicated that they were amenable to surrogacy because of the money it would bring into the family. Some men, like Russell Peters, cushioned the impact of this information by using a jovial tone when communicating it. As I will explore further in the following chapter, talking about compensation and identifying it as a motivation to engage in surrogacy borders on taboo in the US surrogacy community. Therefore, Russell first wanted to assure me that his wife was "not doing it just for the money. She's really *not* doing it just for the money." "However," Russell went on with a big smile on his face and a joking tone, "I don't want to sound greedy, but I'm doing it more for money than she is!" Other men expressed similar sentiments. Douglas Farro, for example, noted that he was pleased with his wife's becoming a surrogate because her fees totaled "a nice sizable amount."

As I noted above, only one woman in my study was engaging in a surrogacy journey without compensation. Other women were open to the idea of an altruistic surrogacy, they told me, but their husbands were not. Sandra Foster, for example, told me that her husband insisted she be paid. She would have "done it for expenses only" (that is, receiving no compensation, only having her expenses paid for) "if only my husband would agree to that."

Surrogates also reported that their husbands were involved in determining their final compensation package. While some women wanted to reduce the amount of the fees they received to save their IPs money, they told me that their husbands were adamant that they receive a particular dollar amount. This was the case with Sandra. Not only did her husband, Thomas, insist that she receive compensation, but she reported that he was adamant that she receive the fee that was standard for her agency. Thomas and other husbands believed that if their wives were to agree to engage in altruistic surrogacy, in which surrogates are not paid, or to accept a lesser amount of money, the women would be cheated out of what was "rightfully theirs." As it was, Thomas argued that the compensation Sandra received "was not nearly enough" for everything she went through.

On surrogate support websites you can read about this notion—that the desire for compensation or a certain fee amount is primarily that of husbands rather than surrogates. Some are skeptical of this notion, arguing that is a convenient position for women to take, allowing them to present themselves as altruistically minded while at the same time receiving the compensation they desire. For example, Sherry Woods said "that husband thing is thrown around" by women who are "try[ing] to pretend they are not" interested in surrogacy because of compensation. She continued: "It's kind of funny, because you always hear surrogates who also talk about, 'Well, I'd do it for nothing but my husband blah, blah, blah.' Really? I don't think so. Maybe they would do it for fairly low [fees]. 'I'd do it for nothing but my husband says it's worth the comp[ensation] and blah, blah.' Well, yeah! Why do it for nothing? The REs get paid, the lawyers get paid. It is providing a service."

Quite a few surrogates told me that they contemplated altruistic surrogacy but that their husbands convinced them not to do it. In discussing this with me, they largely justified bending to their husbands' will on compensation by calling on notions of family sacrifice. This can be seen in Sandra's explanation of why she contracted for the standard fee rather than having an altruistic or reduced fee arrangement, which was her original desire: "I've got to take everyone into consideration there, especially my husband. Considering there's not much more in it for him than that, those extras. He has to put up with me a heck of a lot more than [my IPs] do!"

Evident in Sandra's comments is a sentiment popular in my sample: that surrogacy is a sacrifice for surrogates' families, something that husbands and children have to "put up with." In her study on how class and gender shaped women's work, Sarah Damaske (2011) found similar sentiments of husbands having to endure their wives' employment. Families must endure time away from home and family that surrogacy-related appointments impose, the mood swings surrogates experience due to IVF medication and pregnancy, and the way surrogacy takes over surrogates' lives in terms of the excitement and attention surrogates give to their own journeys and those of others. As will be discussed in depth in the following chapter, because families tolerate surrogacy, compensation becomes a thank-you gift for them. Thus, similar to the decision to pursue surrogacy, compensation was viewed and used not as individual pay for individual work, but as family pay for family work—or rather, family reward for family sacrifice. This can be seen in how surrogates use their compensation. The surrogates in my study indicated that they used it for family-related needs, such as paying off car loans or credit cards, making large purchases for the home, taking their family on a vacation, or putting it into savings for college or retirement. Two women spoke of having or contemplating tummy tucks or breast implants using some of their surrogacy fees, but both jokingly framed those procedures as "family need," saying they were special "gifts" for their husbands.

While compensation can be seen as a real benefit for surrogates and their families, and some men did identify it as what made them agree to surrogacy, most of the men in my study did not speak much about compensation or identify it as what convinced them to accept surrogacy. Rather, they spoke about the joy that surrogacy brought to their wives. For example, Louis Vargas reported his wife's enjoyment of pregnancy and how excited she was by the prospect of surrogacy when she first heard about it. She had been "moping around the house" after the birth of their last child, Louis told me, until she learned about surrogacy. When he told her, "just look into it," he "could just see the glow in her face when she finally found out something like that," because "for some reason she loves being pregnant." Louis appeared to genuinely enjoy his involvement in surrogacy himself. But when I asked him what he enjoyed the most, he replied, "the joy of my wife's, the joy that she gets out of it." He went on: "If she could do it twenty times, I'd let her. I mean, she seems like she's very nice to speak to and everything, but when she's pregnant you really need to come talk to her because you can just see the glow and the happiness in her. So to see her so happy and everything, that was the most I got out of it: to be able to see her as happy as she was." Other husbands told me that they were equally amenable to their wives pursuing surrogacy because of the happiness they knew pregnancy and helping others brought the women. Joel Winmer, for example, let me know that his wife "felt strongly that she always wanted to do [surrogacy]. She liked to do it." Because of this, Joel was "excited for her." "I didn't have a problem with it," he told me, "as long as [the babies] weren't coming home with her, it was fine with me!" This was the position of most husbands in my study. Once they were assured that the surro-babies would share no genetic connection with their wives, they were amenable to surrogacy because they knew their wives would enjoy the process. Many men admired their wives for their surrogacy work. Some spoke of the benefit surrogacy fees would bring their families, but most did not. This is not, of course, a zero-sum game: as I will explore further in the following chapter, surrogates and their husbands can both appreciate the immense pleasure that surrogacy brings to women and desire and insist on compensation.

HUSBANDS' PARTICIPATION

Once husbands agree to surrogacy, not only do they give oral or written consent and sign surrogacy contracts, but they are also expected to participate in the surrogacy process in several other ways. The first involves medical screening and testing. In addition to the psychological evaluation some husbands undergo, many agencies and/or REs (though not all) require any sexual partners (not only legal spouses) to undergo medical screening, usually in the form of blood tests.

The Food and Drug Administration regulates the donation of "human cells, tissues, and cellular and tissue-based products" (HTC/P; 2007). Under these regulations, any parties donating biological matter for the creation and gestation of children must be tested for certain infectious and communicable diseases. IPs using their own gametes and egg and sperm donors are therefore federally required to undergo medical screening. According to the American Society for Reproductive Medicine, though the "FDA does not require screening or testing of gestational carriers for possible transmissible infectious diseases to the fetus," the society "recommends testing of all gestational carriers and their partners within thirty days before embryo transfer to protect the health and interests of all parties involved" (2012a, 1304).

The American Society for Reproductive Medicine recommends that both surrogates and (donating) IPs (but not surrogates' husbands or partners) be tested for "syphilis, gonorrhea, chlamydia, CMV [cytomegalovirus], HIV [human immunodeficiency virus], and hepatitis B and C" (2012b, 15). It also recommends blood typing, Rh factor testing, and screening for "immunity to rubella, rubeola, and varicella" for surrogates, along with a "hysterosalpingo-gram, sonohysterogram, or hysteroscopy" evaluation of the uterine cavity.

Egg and sperm donors (whether IPs themselves or paid or voluntary donors) must be tested because of HTC/P regulations. Gestational surrogates, however, do not donate eggs or tissue. They donate the use of their uteruses, which are not federally regulated. Neither is the social arrangement of gestational surrogacy. Though REs and surrogacy agencies are not federally required to medically test gestational surrogates, the industry standard is to screen women acting as car-riers. All of the women in my study indicated they were screened and tested.

There is greater variation in the testing requirements of different surrogacy agencies and REs offices for husbands and partners. Some agencies and REs refuse to work with women whose husbands will not submit to medical screening, while others do not require any testing for the husbands. Virtually all of the surrogates in my study indicated that their husbands were tested, though several were not. Those surrogates whose husbands were tested were told that this was a requirement of their participation in surrogacy. Most husbands indicated that these tests were not burdensome, though some complained about being "poked and prodded." Most, however, downplayed the invasiveness of their medical testing (for example, saying "it was only a blood test"), juxtaposing it to the more extensive and invasive procedures their wives endured. According to postings on surrogacy message boards, some husbands (though none in my study) refuse medical testing, especially that which involves more invasive testing such as penile swabbing (which is used in testing males for chlamydia and gonorrhea). Those agencies and REs who do require the testing of husbands usually screen for HIV, hepatitis, gonorrhea, syphilis, and human T-cell leukemia virus type 1 (HTLV-1). Many surrogates and their spouses or partners are tested for drug use as well.

Another way husbands are involved in surrogacy is through their abstinence. Surrogates and their sexual partners are asked to refrain from sexual intercourse preceding and following embryo transfers. This contractual obligation is in place to rule out the possibility that the pregnancy might actually be the surrogate's rather than the IPs'. Surrogates are also on "pelvic rest" following the IVF procedure, based on the belief that not disturbing the pelvis will increase the chances that the embryo will adhere to the uterine wall and a pregnancy will occur. For monogamous couples, this means that surrogates' husbands underwent a period of abstinence with each embryo transfer. And because it can take multiple embryo transfers to achieve pregnancy and live birth (and because many surrogates engage in multiple journeys), surrogacy often equates to multiple periods of abstinence over the course of several years.

According to my interviews, the abstinence period requested by REs is usually three weeks per embryo transfer (the week prior to the IVF procedure and the two weeks following the transfer until the pregnancy can be confirmed by a blood test). Many surrogates—and some of their husbands—indicated that they felt more comfortable abstaining for longer periods of time than the medically recommended three weeks. Some extended the period out of concern, anxiety, or superstition about the impact intercourse could have on achieving and sustaining a pregnancy. Other surrogates reported that some of the medications they took for surrogacy led them to feel less than amorous, thus prompting their choice to refrain.

Some surrogates and their partners abstained for a period of four to six weeks with each transfer. For others the self-chosen length of time was longer—for some, months or even more than a year. Ann Beltran, for example, let me know that she and her husband decided to refrain from intercourse for the three months prior to the embryo transfer, "because of all the medications." Once they found out she was pregnant with twins, Ann's husband Bret "had read enough and just was so afraid that something would happen" that they decided to abstain for the entire pregnancy. Ann told me, laughing as she did, that when the intended father found out that they were refraining from sexual intercourse for an entire year because of concerns for his babies, he asked her, "What's your problem?" Ann explained that although they had "never had a problem" due to engaging in sexual intercourse when she was pregnant with her own children, "because it's someone else's child, I think that put a lot on my husband [so] that [he said], 'I don't want anything to happen to these babies, and I don't want to stir anything up or start any labor or whatnot.' So he absolutely was no, not interested—staying away!" Though Ann and her husband had chosen this year-long moratorium on intercourse, it was a challenge for them. Ann characterized both herself and her husband as "troopers," saying a year was "a long time" to renounce sexual intimacy. It was "worth it," however, as both Ann and her husband felt their sacrifice helped them deliver healthy twins to their IPs.

Extended abstinence is also sometimes ordered or recommended by a doctor. Depending on their exact condition, women who experience complications with their surrogacy pregnancies are sometimes put on pelvic rest by their physicians. It is important to note, however, that the majority of women in my study who abstained from sex during surrogacy for long periods of time, like Ann, did so not because it was medically recommended, but because they or their husbands were concerned about the negative impact sexual activity could have on the pregnancy. Some husbands, like Russell Peters, viewed the abstinence as a "minor inconvenience." Others told me that it was more difficult for them to refrain from sex for stretches of time.

Not all surrogates chose to extend the required abstinence period. Some let me know that they simply took the advice of their REs and waited until after the three-week period to commence their regular pattern of intercourse. Others said that pregnancy was a "turn on" for them or their husbands, indicating that sexual activity increased during their surrogacy pregnancies. One of the intended mothers (IMs) in my study, Robin Clark, let me know that her surrogate, who had engaged in multiple surrogacies, informed her that she and her husband enjoyed an active sex life during surrogacy: "She basically said one of the reasons why she liked to be pregnant all the time is because she gets so horny when she's pregnant, and they have sex all the time. So she tells me this when she's pregnant [with my baby]. And I'm thinking, 'That's interesting. The baby is getting bumped around all the time.' Okay. Whoa. And my husband thought it was a little too much information!" Others found sexual intercourse uncomfortable during pregnancy, especially late in the third trimester. For example, Allison Farro, who was twenty-five weeks pregnant when we talked, told me that her husband thought pregnancy was "sexy": "He loves me pregnant. Like the way I am right now? He thinks that's just the most beautiful thing in the world. Which kind of is hard because I feel like an elephant right now! And he's all [giving me bedroom eyes] . . . and I just want to read a book!"

Though some husbands saw abstinence as a sacrifice they made on behalf of surrogacy, quite a few women, like Allison, indicated that they themselves had no difficulty abstaining from sex due to the effects of the hormonal and body changes that come with pregnancy. This is not surprising, as among the possible side effects of the medication used in the medical protocol—which shuts down the menstrual cycle, placing women in what is called medical menopause—are hot flashes, mood swings, nausea, tiredness, depression, and a "decrease in sexual ability or desire" (National Library of Medicine 2011).

Many husbands were intimately familiar with their wives' medical protocols not only due to the deleterious effects on their sex life but because another important way that the husbands of the married surrogates in my study contributed to the surrogacy process was through the administration of medication. Quite a few women let me know that they called on their husbands for help with their medications. As discussed above, IVF surrogacy requires the use of injections. While some of the medications are injected into the abdomen or thigh with small needles, others must be injected into the buttocks with larger needles. Some surrogates can administer all of their own medications, but others find that difficult. Women who asked others to assist them called on family members, usually a husband or a daughter. These injectables are prescribed for daily use and therefore require a consistent helper for those needing assistance. As Molly Hughes told me, "you've got to have somebody there every single night to give you your shot."

Many husbands and other family members were initially quite nervous about being able to safely and correctly administer the injections. This task was sometimes difficult given the body's physical reaction to so many injections (surrogates spoke of being bruised black and blue) and sometimes because of the circumstances in which the injections took place. For example, Keri Woltz, who was between fourteen and twenty-five years of age when her mother was on her five surrogacy journeys (for which she had eighteen embryo transfer cycles), spoke of administering her mother's medication: "I remember how bruised she used to be. She used to be black and blue—her thighs and her stomach were just one big bruise. It was crazy. I remember having to stop at truck stop bathrooms in the stalls when we went on vacation. And I was giving her shots in the stall. And people were trying to peek!"

Some family members were so afraid of needles that they refused to participate. For example, Tina Vargas gave herself all of her shots because her husband could not handle the needles (he told me this while also joking that he could not change diapers). Other family members were panicky about correctly administering the injections but persisted despite their nerves. For example, Russell

Peters let me know that he had to "give all the shots, which obviously I had never done before." Russell had been administering the shots for years when I met him, as his wife, Erin, was on her fourth surrogacy journey. "I like to think I've gotten better at it as I've done it how many different times," Russell said. When I asked him how he felt about giving Erin her shots, he told me, laughing: "I feel like I don't know what I'm doing. And even though she says 'you're not going to hurt me,' I don't want to do the wrong thing. So it's not *that* big of a deal, but I'm happy when it's over with and I don't have to give the shots anymore!"

This was the general sentiment of most family members who were involved in this aspect of surrogacy. Not only were they happy with the cessation of their nursing duties, but they could set aside their anxieties about any immediate negative medical repercussions surrogacy might entail once their wives or mothers completed their journeys. These anxieties were not limited to injuring the women during injections. Some husbands also reported more general fears about the possibility of complications arising during IVF-related procedures or pregnancy and birth and long-term negative health impacts that their wives might experience due to the medications they took.

Concerns about Health and Safety

After concerns regarding biological connections between their wives and surro-babies, concerns for their wives' health was the second major reason husbands were apprehensive about their wives participating in surrogacy. Unlike concerns about the genetic relatedness between surrogates and surro-babies, however, husbands' concerns regarding the health and safety of their wives were never resolved and were ongoing throughout their journeys.

When Joel Winmer discussed his wife's first surrogacy journey, which resulted in the birth of twins, he said: "Of course there's always concern for her health, especially initially with the first twins and her not carrying twins before and some of the complications she had there, that was definitely a concern. But everything first and foremost has been for her health. And as long as she was healthy and okay with it, then I had no problems [with her being a surrogate]." Treena, Joel's wife, was like many surrogates (and nonsurrogate pregnant women) in experiencing minor complications with her pregnancies. The most potentially serious condition during Treena's two surrogacy pregnancies was placenta previa, in which the placenta lies too low in the uterus, either partially or totally covering the opening in the cervix. This condition was Joel's "biggest concern" because of the severe bleeding it can cause. "If she starts bleeding," he noted, "she can bleed out very quickly." Like many husbands, Joel felt the need to stay consistently vigilant about his wife's physical safety during pregnancy: "So that's my only concern with all the pregnancies. And so far, knock on wood, everything has gone smooth[ly]. It's just one of those things to keep in the back of your mind—to watch things and don't take anything for granted at that point."

Husbands' concerns about the health and safety of their surrogate wives were not unwarranted. Many of participants in my study experienced some sort of pregnancy, birth, or postpartum medical complication during their experiences working as a surrogate. Some conditions, such as placenta previa, severe pre-eclampsia, or HELLP syndrome (which, as discussed in the previous chapter, caused Amanda Wagner to have a stillbirth), were potentially life threatening; others were less serious.

These complications were disconcerting for surrogates' husbands and children, not only because they posed a threat to the health and safety of their loved ones, but because they often affected the ability of surrogates to participate in regular family life. This was especially evident when surrogates were put on doctor-ordered bed rest.

BED REST

Most women were on bed rest directly following embryo transfer. This type of bed rest was not of an emergency nature; it was not ordered out of medical concern, but due to physicians' beliefs that it would aid pregnancy. Not all REs subscribe to this traditional view, however. A few women in my study were allowed to rise directly after the procedure and carry on as normal. Most, however, had to lie flat on their backs for several hours, with many then having to remain relatively immobile for several days. Quite a few of the women in my study spent three or four days in bed following a transfer.

Transfer-related bed rest was anticipated and, therefore, surrogates made appropriate plans for their families. Depending on their location, embryo transfer procedures can require travel for surrogates. This was the case for many of my participants, who then stayed at hotels paid for by their IPs. Some agencies ask for no visitors during bed rest (sometimes limiting that restriction to only those visitors who would keep the surrogate from resting); others had no restrictions. Surrogates who worked with agencies and REs who did not discourage visitors often took their families with them on transfer day, staying at a hotel and enjoying a "minivacation" of TV-viewing marathons and take-out food while their children swam in the hotel pool with their husbands. Those surrogates able to take their children spoke of those hotel visits as enjoyable times for their families. Their children and husbands did as well. Keri Woltz, for example, spoke with fondness of accompanying her mother: "I remember going, and then she had to be on bed rest for three days afterward, and we could sit in a hotel room and have room service and just lay in bed and watch TV. That was the best time! I enjoyed it! It was fun. It was like all fun and games to me. I was like, 'Whoo-hoo!'" Molly Hughes spoke of transfer bed rest in similar terms.

Her children, she told me, "love it. [My IM] always gets us a hotel with a pool, and they just spend three days in the pool. So what are they going to complain about? And mom can't get off the bed and do anything. We have fun. It's almost like a minivacation." Others indicated that transfer-related bed rest was an enjoyable break from the hustle of everyday life and a time of great anticipation as they looked forward to the surrogacy journey. Ann Beltran, for example, told me that she loved the three days of bed rest she experienced following her embryo transfer: "For me [best rest] is fabulous because I never get to lay in bed for three days! Are you kidding!? [laughing] I enjoyed it!! And [my IPs] sent flowers and stuff like that."

Those unable to take their young children with them on the transfer trip, while equally excited about surrogacy, often found the time away from their families stressful. They indicated that their children missed them or that they had to miss out on family events, which they found upsetting. Even those surrogates who spent bed rest at home sometimes had to miss out on family events—sometimes even events occurring in their own homes. For example, though Ann loved her rest (and the flowers), she was not able to enjoy her son's birthday celebration with her family because she was resting in her bedroom. "And everybody was out here singing," she told me as we sat in her living room, "and I was in my bedroom."

Sometimes the family events that surrogates are unable to attend due to transfer and the accompanying bed rest are important ones in the life of their families: a graduation, a family reunion, a school event. Laurel Molza, for example, had to miss an important performance of her husband, Dwight: "And it just happened to be the same weekend that I was on bed rest. And it was just such a phenomenal, huge weekend for him. And I'm here [at home]. It's just one of those things. You hate to call it a job, but it's part of the job sometimes. You make those sacrifices. That was hard on both of us because it was such a monumental moment for him that I missed." Dwight let me know that though he was sad that his wife could not attend his big event, both he and Laurel understood their sacrifice as necessary. This was just one of the "sacrifices you make" for surrogacy, according to my participants.

It was more challenging for the young children of surrogates to adopt that outlook. Quite a few women reported that their children found the time apart from their mothers difficult. Dawn Rudge, for example, let me know that the time away from her family for her transfer was a "big issue" for Ivy, her seven-year-old daughter. Ivy had wanted to be part of the whole surrogacy experience and felt as though she were "missing out" on an important part of the process when she was not allowed to join her mother on the transfer trip. She also simply missed her mother, as did her two siblings.

This issue of separation from the family and missing family events was even more problematic for women who experienced medical complications resulting in doctor-ordered bed rest. While most experienced post-transfer bed rest, more than 40 percent of my surrogate participants experienced doctor-ordered bed rest due to medical complications. For several women, the issue necessitating the bed rest was serious enough that they had to be hospitalized. Cindy Woltz, for example, had severe bleeding due to placenta previa with one of her surrogacies, the same condition experienced by Treena Winmer, in which the placenta lies too low in the uterus. Unlike Treena, for Cindy the condition led to serious complications and bed rest in the hospital.

Diagnosed at twenty-eight weeks gestation during an amniocentesis procedure in which a high-resolution ultrasound was performed, Cindy was immediately put on bed rest at home. She woke a week later in the middle of the night, hemorrhaging severely. Cindy rushed to the bathroom with "blood all over" her, "almost spraying out." She screamed for her husband, Chuck, who helped her undress so she could shower (she "didn't want to go to the emergency room just covered in blood" she told me). Before they left for the hospital, Cindy and Chuck woke their high-school-age daughter, Keri. It was 3:00 A.M., and "blood was all over the carpet. On the bed—it was everywhere." Chuck quickly got Cindy to the hospital and, though it was the middle of the night and she had school the next day, Keri cleaned her mother's blood from the bathroom and bedroom.

I asked Keri, a young adult when we spoke, what that experience had been like for her. Keri replied, "I was really afraid that something had happened to her." At that point, though, her mother was on her third surrogacy, and Keri had experienced other episodes of her mother bleeding and having to deal with serious complications. "As far as seeing the blood," Keri went on, "we had dealt with the bleeding so many times before that it was just kind of like, 'Oh wow! This is kind of a lot. All right, I'll clean it up.'"

Cindy remained in the hospital "on complete bed rest" for the next four weeks, "hemorrhaging all the time":

> I had two showers the whole month. The rest were sponge baths. I wasn't allowed up to use the toilet. [I was] completely in bed. I had eight catheters during the time I was there. I was always on an IV. They started looking for veins in my legs because my veins were all blown. I was on every kind of drug because what would happen was I'd start hemorrhaging and that would spark labor. So then they'd have to try and stop the contractions because if my cervix started opening . . . they kept telling me, "You can die in five minutes. You can bleed out in five minutes." So my room was right across from the OR. And I just stayed in the hospital.

She delivered "a day shy of thirty-three weeks" via emergency cesarean section due to a severe hemorrhage. She was in the hospital for just over a month.

Though Cindy's story is dramatic in terms of its severity, it contains several elements common to the surrogacy experiences of husbands and children. Like Cindy, all of the women who had experienced doctor-ordered bed rest spoke of the problems this created for their families. Jessica Klein, for example, experienced a subchorionic hematoma (bleeding that occurs inside the placenta or in the membrane surrounding the placenta) and spent five weeks in bed at her home. She spoke of the challenges she faced trying to mother her two young children, Clay and Skyler, and how her husband, Aaron—like Cindy's husband, Chuck—had to take over the household duties:

> It was awful being on bed rest. Clay was three, so Skyler was seven. She's going to school. Clay went to preschool. It was hard. I couldn't do anything. I'm just in bed, and Clay would say, "I want Mommy to tuck me in. I want Mommy to kiss me." He's just a little boy, not understanding why is mom just laying in bed? I couldn't sit up and do Skyler's hair. I had to lay back. I couldn't give her a ponytail. She had to squat down next to the bed. Just simple motherly things you do every day I couldn't do. And it was very frustrating. And Aaron had to go to work and come home and do everything. . . . But it was awful. But I knew I had to do it, and I was just so thankful when I got to get up again.

While Jessica's and Cindy's experiences with bed rest varied in their severity, they both highlight common issues. For Jessica and Cindy and other surrogates in my study, the medical demands of surrogacy and the complications that can arise sometimes affect the ability of surrogates to participate in normal family life.

Family Time

Surrogacy was a time-consuming process for many women. Not only did it require multiple visits to agency, RE, and obstetrician-gynecologist (OB/GYN) offices, but it often involved visits with IPs, other surrogates, and attendance at support group meetings and social events. Some new surrogates were surprised by the amount of time involved. Screening, testing, transfer, and monitoring appointments dominate the start-up of surrogacy journeys, and visits with OBs become more frequent as birth draws near. Even uncomplicated pregnancies and births affected what was often referred to as "family time." Surrogates also let me know that they found surrogacy a tremendous amount of fun and enjoyment, with it often coming to dominate their "down time" through social interactions with other surrogates and spending time online reading blogs and visiting surrogacy message boards. As Deanna Meer told me, "it consumes your life, it really does. I wouldn't change it, I love it, but it does—it consumes your life."

Many women indicated that in their homes, they were the ones primarily responsible for child care and housework. This was especially true for the twelve women who did not work outside of the home. While just over 60 percent of the women who spoke with me had outside employment (which they continued during their surrogacy journeys), they also reported a "second shift" burden of child care and housework after they returned home from work (Hochschild 1989). The research on the division of labor in the home indicates that the participants in my study were not unlike many women in the United States, who shoulder much of the housework regardless of their participation in paid labor (Bianchi et al. 2006; Hansen 2005; Maume et al. 2010).

There was a theme that ran throughout my interviews: surrogacy caused problems related to child care and housework. This was especially true for women with children under the age of five. At the time of their first surrogacy journey, nineteen out of my thirty-one participants had children younger than five in the home. The remaining twelve participants had children in elementary school or junior high school, with the oldest child of three-quarters of those women under the age of ten.

The issue of child care cropped up when women had appointments that took them outside the home. While for some of those visits, children and families were welcome or tolerated; for others, as Rosalyn Whelan noted, young children were not allowed to accompany their mothers. Rosalyn explained that because of this she arranged for her one-year-old son, Cooper, to attend an in-home day care whenever she had medical appointments: "I had to [put Cooper in day care] from the beginning because it's so many appointments and it's very frowned upon in the infertility world to bring your child anywhere near an infertility clinic. You don't do that. Some people do, but it's just like—it's just not—a lot of people that are there, I guess—you don't know what they're going through. You don't know at what point in their struggle they're in." Sensitive to the emotional needs of others, Rosalyn, a recently separated single mother, found that paid help worked best when she had her RE appointments. Other surrogates unable to take their children with them, especially at the beginning of the surrogacy journey (which involves visits to the RE's office), also arranged for paid child care, while some called on older children, their husbands, or members of their extended family and friends to help care for their young children so they could attend surrogacy appointments.

Some surrogates, but not all, received an allowance or reimbursement from the IPs for child care. Some women were like Amber Castillo, who let me know that she had to schedule her surrogacy appointments carefully to coincide with times that her husband or sister were available to watch her children due to the fact that she did not have enough disposable income to cover the cost of child care for every appointment. Some women avoided paid help not only due to a lack of funds. Some surrogates had child care reimbursement stipulated in their surrogacy contracts, but refused to access it because they wanted to save their IPs money. Instead, they called on their family members and friends to watch their children when they needed child-care assistance. Other women, like many American parents, preferred family care over paid care (Hansen 2005, 6). One such participant in my study was Jessica Klein. A stay-at-home mother, Jessica told me, "I hate leaving [my children] with babysitters, which is why I've been home for almost eleven years." Jessica went on, however, to tell me that she has used paid child care "a couple times." "Whatever is going to work for the pregnancy and for my family," she said, "is what's best for me."

One of the ways women structure their journeys to help mitigate adding surrogacy appointments to already complicated family calendars and caregiving needs is by scheduling their surrogacy journeys, as much as possible, around the academic calendar for their school-age children. Because she disliked using babysitters, this was a strategy used by Jessica, who had to travel several hours each way to attend appointments. She explained what her schedule would look like on appointment days: "I would go [to appointments] when they were in school. I'd drop them off at school, make my appointment three hours from that time, do my appointment, have lunch real quick or grab something, and get back to pick them up."

This allowed Jessica and other women to plan for the bulk of their time away from their families to occur during the school day, which made things easier on their children and, if the women were married, their spouses. Keeping life relatively normal for their kids while fulfilling their surrogacy duties, although a balancing act, was a stated goal of many of the participants in my study. Dawn Rudge, for example, let me know that she preferred her journeys to occur during the school year. She explained: "Mainly it's my kids, and if the transfer was during the school year—I didn't want anybody to be put out or [for the process] to be any more traumatic on my kids. Traumatic might not be the right word, but I wanted life to be as close to normal as it could be."

While several women let me know that surrogacy and pregnancy had no effect on their ability to keep life "normal," most said that the journey affected their day-to-day home life. Surrogacy work not only involved time away from the home, necessitating making child-care arrangements for young children, but it also shaped women's ability to keep up with their normal housework.

Surrogacy can be physically and emotionally draining. The administration of surrogacy medication and its effects, for example, can cause tiredness and frequent mood changes, which altered the regular family routine for my participants (National Library of Medicine 2011). Sometimes surrogates were unable to keep up with their regular household tasks due to the demands of surrogacy or the exhaustion that can accompany IVF and pregnancy. This was especially a problem for women experiencing pregnancy complications, especially those on bed rest. But women who had no complications also spoke of slowing down and being unable to keep up with housework, especially as their pregnancies neared their conclusion.

Some surrogates have money in their compensation packages dedicated to hiring a housecleaner, while others ask their family members to pick up the slack. As with child care, some women felt uncomfortable hiring someone to clean their home for them, and others did not want their IPs to experience that added financial burden. Husbands and children, especially older children, therefore often found themselves performing housework and child care that they normally were not responsible for so that surrogates could take care of their surrogacy responsibilities or rest.

Surrogacy not only affects women's ability to perform housekeeping and child care, it can also affect the quality of interactions surrogates have with their families and the general mood in the household. Most participants indicated that at times they felt that medication negatively affected their temperament. Some referred to one of the surrogacy drugs as "loopy Lupron." Ann Beltran, for example, explained that the medication made her moody and short-tempered with her children. "Just a lot of the hot flashes," she said, "and you're a little more angry. Little things that probably just bother you, you're a little more emotional about. And tears will come. That part is kind of hard, and I'm sure the kids were probably looking at me most of the time like, 'You're nuts!' And yeah, so that was hard for them."

The strict medical protocol also restricted movement for surrogates' families. For example, Kelly Russo, one of the four single women in my study, spoke of having to forgo outings, like a trip to SeaWorld, because of the demands of the medical protocol: "There's a lot of times when I couldn't go do something because I had to have a shot at this time. So I wanted to take my daughter to SeaWorld with a friend of mine. But my friend refused to do the shot, and I was like, 'Well, I can't do it myself so I can't go.' I had to be where my daughter's nanny was—who gave me my shots—at 6:00 every night. So I had to make sacrifices." Both the husbands who spoke with me and the surrogates in my study let me know that both they and their families sacrificed "family time" for surrogacy. Molly Hughes, for example, said: "This whole process had monopolized a lot of our time as far as my kids are concerned. Luckily I'm a stay-at-home mom, but there's just certain things that we couldn't do because I was pregnant. They [her children] get free Six Flags tickets every year from school and we go, and I didn't get to go this year. They went with my husband and another friend. So there's just little things like that that because of the surrogacy we didn't get to do."

Such sacrifices did not always sit well with husbands and children. Some family members, especially children, were sometimes unhappy with their mother's mood swings, the time away from the family that surrogacy exacts, or the extra labor they were forced to contribute. In my interview with Tina Vargas, for example, she let me know how much assistance she received from her husband, Louis, and her older daughter, Morgan, who was then fourteen. Tina and Louis adhered to a traditional gendered division of labor in the home, which was strained by surrogacy and necessitated Morgan's assistance. As a stay-at-home mother and primary caregiver to two teenage children, two elementary-school-age children, and an elderly mother with health issues, Tina needed Morgan's help with day-to-day housework, child care, and elder care to be a surrogate. This was especially difficult during the first three months of a journey when Tina felt the negative effects of IVF medication, often knocking her out for the day and putting her on the couch. Morgan was often called on to watch the younger children and assist with her grandmother. Louis let me know that Morgan was quite resistant to the idea of her mother's completing another surrogacy because of the increase in work around the house that would mean for her. Louis explained:

> Morgan has already told my wife she don't want her doing any more [surrogacies]. She said it's been a toll on her body and also it's because she's having to kick in and help out a lot with the kids, with the kitchen, with the cleaning. Especially once my wife gets into a certain part of her pregnancy, we don't let her do as much. So Morgan really is happy and she loves the babies, she has pictures of them in her phone and all that—but when we go to let her know her mom's going to do it one more time, she was like, "Oh no. No more."

As Louis's comments indicate, according to their parents, the children of surrogates had complex feelings about their mothers' participation in surrogacy and how it shaped family time. As Keri Woltz told me, "a lot of the time" growing up with a surrogate mother "sucked because she was on the phone for five hours straight talking about surrogate stuff. And we'd all give her a hard time about it; throwing stuff at her in the background. It did consume a lot of her time, but I'm happy that she did it."

Surrogates' Children

Surrogates' children are an important part of the surrogacy equation. At the beginning of the process, children serve as markers that enable women to work as surrogates for agencies, since women must be mothers to be hired. But the existence of those children also shapes the choices women make and the experiences they have serving as surrogates.

The impact of surrogacy on the lives of their children was an initial concern for many of the surrogates in my study. Many women indicated that their children were excited about the prospect of their families participating in surrogacy but initially confused about the identity of the potential surro-babies. This was a deep concern of my participants, and they worked in various ways to address the confusion. All of my participants indicated that they were truthful with their children about surrogacy (in age-appropriate ways), as is the industry standard. As Treena Winmer put it, "we never sugarcoated or hid anything from them."

Most of the women with young children—who made up the majority of my sample—reported that they shared a version of the "broken tummy" story to explain gestational surrogacy to their children. April Palmer, for example, told her two young daughters that her IM's "tummy was broken, and that the doctor was going to put her baby in my tummy until it was ready to be out, and then it would go to the mom." April said that this simple explanation worked well: "They got it. They never really questioned it. Kids are really accepting of things in a way that adults are not." All of my other participants also reported that their children who were old enough to do so understood surrogacy and accepted the arrangement.

Like April, when talking with their children other surrogates explicitly framed surrogacy as a gift that they were giving to their IPs. Their "IPs need help and Mommy is going to give it," was the refrain. Deidre Richards, for example, reported that when she was pregnant with twins for her IPs, Damian and Pauline, she told her five-year-old son, "I think it would make Damian and Pauline really happy if we could give them these babies since they don't have any." This framing of surrogacy as a gift was an important strategy to help young children understand surrogacy and their own relationship to the surro-babies.

A challenge for many surrogates was the fact that their young children did not have a working knowledge of reproduction. Quite a few women, therefore, let me know that surrogacy was a catalyst for talking with their children about human sexuality and reproduction. Molly Hughes, for example, shared a common dilemma surrogates face: for many, the first experience their young children have witnessing pregnancy close-up is via IVF and surrogacy. Molly let me know, laughing as she did, that her "kids have not [got] a good view of how pregnancy happens." Their understanding of human reproduction involves "shots and shots and shots and pills and pills and you go into the doctor's office and you find out two weeks later, did it work?" "It's so hard," Molly went on, "because they've got a skewed vision of how pregnancy happens. My kids think you get pregnant by injections!"

Several surrogates let me know that the "birds and bees talk" was accelerated in their homes due to their participation in surrogacy. Dawn Rudge's seven-year-old daughter, for example, "needed information and wanted to know what was going on." Dawn continued: "For her, we had to get a little more detailed than I thought I would need to. And we had to break it down, and we talked about eggs and sperm and really explained to her that this is not her brother and sister, and this is why."

Helping their children understand reproduction was a strategy surrogates used to prepare their children for the birth and relinquishment of surro-babies. Rhonda Chapman, for example, spoke of needing to educate her five-year-old son "on reproduction the normal way, starting out talking about the bees and flowers." Rhonda felt she needed to "kind of ease him into that and start out with how it's usually done. And then get into the different ways." The goal was a basic understanding of reproduction, leading into the fact that the children his mother was bearing were not his siblings. Rhonda's strategy was successful, as her son "never ever thought it [*sic*] was a brother and sister. He always knew."

Instilling a "correct understanding" of surrogacy in children old enough to comprehend pregnancy and birth, especially those children who had experienced the birth of a sibling, was an important strategy for most surrogates. Some women did not have to concern themselves with this issue. Their children were young enough that they had little or no comprehension of the events swirling around their lives. This was the case with Sandra Foster, who had two children at the time of her first journey. When I asked Sandra what her children thought of surrogacy, she replied: "Well, my kids were really young then, too. My daughters were five and two, I think. And so Ariel had no clue what was going on, she's the little one. And Becca is just drawing pictures and giving them to everybody, which is what five-year-olds do. And so it wasn't really an issue with the kids."

Women with older children indicated that they were frank and honest with their children about surrogacy, coaching them on particular understandings of surrogacy. This can be seen in the exchange Leah Spalding let me know that she had with her seven-year-old daughter, Cassidy:

> I'm pretty honest with my daughter. I talk to her about it, and she doesn't really understand. I mean, she's only seven. But I told her, "Cassidy, how do you feel about me having a baby for someone else?" She's like, "Are you going to give away your baby, Mama?" And I'm like, "Oh, no, no, no. It's going to be the mom's egg and the dad's sperm, but they can't hold it because mom's tummy is broken, so they asked me if I could hold it for them." And she's like, "That's cool!" And she's like, "You're going to give it away?" And I'm like, "I'm not really going to give it away. I'm just babysitting for a while." And she's like, "Well, okay. After you're done can you have one for us?" And I'm like [laughing], "I'm not sure. But I'll think about it."

Leah's strategy was similar to that of other women in my study who sought to normalize surrogacy for their children. According to my interviews, this approach was usually successful. While some children were uninterested in surrogacy (Allison Farro, for example, told me that her nine-year-old daughter Jordyn "was kind of like, 'whatever,'" when she tried to explain surrogacy to her), none of my participants reported their children were hostile or upset about the pregnancy. Most were similar to the children of Josephine Maselli. "It is a normal thing for them," Josephine told me:

> And they understand it. It was never a question of whose baby it was. They just understand that I am just helping. We don't hide anything like that from them. Every time I've gone, they've known that it hasn't worked. They've

looked at the pictures—each time you get a little picture of the embryos they put in. They've looked at them and know that that is what went inside me. So I don't know if they really understand why it's not working or what exactly happens to the embryos. But for their age levels they understand it and accept it very well.

In fact, surrogacy was so normalized for the children that they spoke quite openly and frankly about their mothers' participation in surrogacy. Treena Winmer told me that her children "say it exactly the way that it is: 'My mom is a surrogate, and she's carrying twins for a couple.' They say it exactly the way it is. They're able to understand it. When that's what they've known and it's not a taboo thing, they don't treat it as such." Like Treena, the other participants in my study indicated that because surrogacy was normalized for their children, they sometimes created awkward situations for their parents. April Palmer, for example, said that during her surrogacy when she was out in public, visibly pregnant, with her children they would often be asked, "Are you getting a brother or a sister?" April told me her children would then respond with a simple "'no' and turn and walk away! And I'd have to explain. Because to them it was just—it is what it is. 'No, I'm not getting a brother or sister.' But I'm pregnant out to here!"

Children also shared the fact that their mother was a surrogate with other people in their lives: their friends, teachers, and classmates; and people at church and camp. Deidre Richards, for example, told me a story about her young son, Trevor, educating a member of their church about his mother's surrogacy:

One of the ladies at church said something to [my son] because she hadn't heard, I guess, that I was carrying for another couple. And during Sunday school she said something to Trevor about him being a big brother: "Are you excited about your mommy having another little brother or sister for you?" And Trevor said, "They're not ours!" [laughing] And she just kind of laughed because Trevor is just too outgoing anyway. She's like, "Oh, Trevor, you're being so silly." He goes, "No! I'm serious. They're not ours. Mommy is having those babies for Damian and Pauline. They're Damian and Pauline's babies."

Deidre was quite proud of Trevor, especially as his rendition was correct and did not cause an awkward social situation with the woman at church. In fact, the church member approached Deidre after the service and said to her, "I just want to let you know I think that's great that you're being a surrogate for them. You've trained your son well, because he's already telling everybody that they're not yours!" Molly Hughes shared a similar story regarding her ten-year-old daughter, Nina. After school one day, Molly asked Nina, "So do your friends know that I'm pregnant? And do they know about the surrogacy, what it is and all that?" Nina told her mother, "Mom, it's all we talk about at lunch." Though Nina "didn't know any words or lingo or anything," she told her classmates: "They took this part from the mom and the dad, and my mom's just carrying it and she's going to give it back to them."

Sometimes children's sharing of information, like Nina's with her classmates, would cause misunderstandings, especially if the children did not fully divulge all of the important information. Douglas Farro shared such a story involving his daughter and her school. His daughter was "talking about" the pregnancy at school but somehow "impl[ied]" that she was going to have siblings." Though Douglas and his wife had been "as clear as can be 'this is what's going on,'" the teachers and administrators did not understand that this was a surrogacy situation, which caused them some awkwardness at the school.

Douglas's story highlights a dilemma faced by other families in my study. Women in my study let me know that they and their husbands were cautious about to whom they divulge information about surrogacy but that their children readily shared details with anyone in their social worlds. So while the children reportedly have good working understandings of surrogacy, it is clear that some of them do not understand the larger social context surrounding surrogacy, which includes stigma. Indicative of this was the experience of Ann Beltran's children. On her second surrogacy journey, Ann began to experience negative reactions from people in her church and school-based social circles. People began ignoring her and talking behind her back. She found out that some people were questioning her motives and saying, "Oh it's terrible what she's doing to her children!" and "Why would you do that again to your children?"

Ann was devastated by the loss of support in her community. She was particularly upset when people began avoiding her children. According to Ann, her children understood they were being treated badly. It was obvious, she said. However, her children did not make the connection between the fact that their mother was a surrogate and this new behavior from their former friends and families in their church and school. "I always found it funny," Ann told me, "that my children could explain the whole IVF procedure and everything that happened, and they had no clue." Instead, her children "knew everything about [surrogacy] and they were proud of it." They simply thought that other people were behaving strangely.

To Ann's children and the other children of surrogates in my study, surrogacy was a normal part of their social world. Keri Woltz, for example, whose mother completed five journeys, told me that growing up with her mother being a surrogate was "kind of just the usual, 'Oh yeah, she's had babies for other people.'" Keri and her older sister experienced some negative reactions in high school because "a lot of people disagree[d] with it." However, other people were supportive, and so "it was always kind of a cool thing to tell people." Though others thought it was a "big deal," Keri "just kind of accepted it as a regular part of our life."

FAMILY CONTACT: SURROGATES,
THEIR HUSBANDS, KIDS, AND IPS

The children of the surrogates in my study had varying relationships with their mothers' IPs. These relationships were highly dependent on the relationship the surrogate herself had with the IPs, the geographical and social distance between the families, IPs' and surrogates' family members' individual interest in cultivating connections, and the involvement level of the family in surrogacy more generally. Some families established close connections with the IPs, participating in social events together and coming to think of each other as relatives of a sort. For other families, interactions with IPs were limited to surrogacy-related appointments, which sometimes involved only adults and not the surrogates' children. Still others had little or no interaction with IPs. All of the surrogates in my study indicated that their family members had at least met (or, for those new to the process, were scheduled to meet) at least one of their IPs. The majority of the women indicated that their husbands or partners and their children had participated in at least one social event with their IPs. Most had experienced multiple interactions.

Integrating the concept of IPs into children's understanding of their mothers' pregnancies was an important strategy used by women in my study for both distancing their families from the surro-babies and ensuring that children did not think about the babies as siblings. Almost all surrogates introduced their children to their IPs, with many having multiple interactions. Those interactions helped to solidify the idea that the babies were not their siblings and, instead, belonged to the IPs. April Palmer shared this idea when talking about the interactions her daughters had with her IPs, Kip and Virginia: "Through the pregnancy we had dinners and [my kids] sometimes were able to go to doctor's appointments with us. We did a couple of social things like SeaWorld, and they came to the kids' birthday parties and that sort of thing. So yeah, [my children] knew [the IPs] definitely through the process. I think that helps. Because it was always Kip and Virginia's baby."

The relationship between a surrogate's family and her IPs often begins with adult-only interactions involving the IPs, the surrogate, and her husband. Husbands and IPs often meet during the matching process. While some surrogates talk with potential IPs via phone or e-mail prior to face-to-face meetings, most of the husbands in my study indicated that their first interaction with IPs was at the "match meeting," during which IPs meet the surrogate for the first time. Some agencies have a fairly structured and ritualized process for that meeting, having it occur at the surrogacy agency office or in a public space such as a restaurant and overseen by an agency employee, often the counselor or the agency owner. Many agencies encourage surrogates' spouses to attend; some require them to be present. Most of the husbands in my study indicated that they wanted to attend as both they and their wives see husbands as central players in the surrogacy arrangement—or at least in the decision to pursue surrogacy and chose the IPs. For some husbands in my study, the match meeting and the birth were their primary face-to-face interactions with the IPs during their wives' journeys. Most husbands in my study, however, had more contact with IPs.

Medical appointments were another important point of contact between IPs and husbands. Many husbands of the surrogates in my study attended medical appointments with their wives, chauffeuring them to the visits and, in some cases, accompanying them into the examination rooms (others waited in the lobby or, if it was a quick visit, in the car). Treena Winmer let me know that her husband, Joel, "has gone to every appointment that I've had. He hasn't missed anything, he won't miss anything." Her IPs also attended all of the appointments. Joel let me know that the IPs "were very, very active. If it wasn't both of them, somebody was at every single appointment through the different doctors and the big appointments—they were both at the sonogram to find out the sex of the kids. I don't know that they could have been any more active throughout the pregnancy. They were just as active as had it been his wife carrying the child." These doctor's visits were opportunities to help solidify friendly connections between Joel and the IPs.

Joel's interactions with the IPs were similar to those of the husbands of other surrogates in my study. Joel and the IPs met at the match meeting, interacted at doctor's appointments, "and then there was a couple dinners just for no specific reason, just dinners with the family." Joel continued: "And then after the delivery we still kept active with them on some things, with the [surro-babies'] birthdays. A couple holidays they'd come over, and we'd go there and have little cookouts." As the surro-babies got older, family interactions began to diminish. Joel's wife, Treena, continued to have some contact with the IM, mostly via e-mail, but Joel had none. Neither Joel nor Treena indicated any upset feelings about the decrease of their contact with the IPs. Joel noted: "We left everything up to them, whatever they were comfortable with, we were open." Joel summarized his experience with surrogacy and with that particular couple by saying, "It was a very neat situation." He enjoyed his time getting to know the IPs and was tremendously proud of his wife for having served as their surrogate.

Joel was an active "surrogate's husband" during the journey. Treena let me know that Joel's commitment and involvement was important: "It's kind of like you either commit to all of it or you don't. You need that support system on both sides [both husbands and wives]. And he's fully committed." Though Joel was a full participant, as a husband he was a secondary player. Treena and the IM made arrangements for the get-togethers, maintained regular contact, and were the people who interacted the most with each other; Joel happily went along for the ride. The Winmers' experiences, which were representative of those of most other participants in my study, are similar to the gendered division of what

Micaela di Leonardo calls "kin work" that can be found in many families, with women assuming responsibility for connecting family members with each other (1987, 442–43).

Like the Winmers, most surrogate families had friendly interactions with their IPs during their journeys, characterized by several social get-togethers that included children and online contact that was mainly between IMs and surrogates, with a gradual reduction in contact following the birth of the surro-babies. Many surrogates in my study reported that they were coached by their agencies and counselors to anticipate a change in the content and form of interaction they had with their IPs after the surro-babies were born. Surrogates were also encouraged to allow IPs to determine how much contact the families would have with one another after the birth.

But other families in my study were different, either becoming exceptionally close to their IPs and continuing to have positive, fulfilling relations with them after the birth of the babies, or having a falling-out with their IPs. The Klein family, discussed in chapter 4, for example, established a familial-like bond with their first IP couple, Gia and Charles. Several years after the birth of her surro-twins, Hope and Milo, Jessica explains her family's current relationship with the IP family as a close one: "I get to keep [babysit for] Hope and Milo," Jessica told me, "and we go spend the night with them. We go on vacations together."

This close relationship helped Jessica's two young children, especially her daughter Skyler, come to accept the surrogacy. Jessica explained that Skyler, who was seven when her mother was pregnant with Hope and Milo, initially had "a hard time" when she found out one of the twins was a girl, because "she wants a sister so bad." Jessica and her husband explained to Skyler that they would not be having more children. They told her: "If we have another baby, God might give us a boy. [And then] we're not going to have a fourth just to see who can try to [give you] a sister. That's why we have friends." "Once she got over that," Jessica told me, "then she was fine." Jessica added that Skyler now "calls Hope her "surro-sister, because that's as close as she's ever getting to a sister!"

Jessica's son, Clay, on the other hand, who was three at the time, was confused about who he was in relation to the babies. Clay repeatedly asked Jessica, "Well, what am I?" He understood that "he's not the big brother," Jessica explained, so he would ask, "What am I?" Jessica would respond, "You're the big friend."

Jessica was happy with the relationship that her family had with Gia and Charles, especially the bonds her children have developed with them. They know that Hope and Milo "are not our babies. But they're our friends, and we get to see them whenever we want. So they're fine with it." The entire family, Jessica told me, has "a very close relationship with Gia and Charles now." The continuing contact is "so rewarding because as a surrogate I get to see everything [I've] worked for all this time, hands on. I couldn't ask for anything better than the way we did it."

The Vargas family was the second family in my study who came to think of one set of their IPs as family members. Louis and Tina were godparents to the surro-twins Tina birthed, and the families have continued frequent contact with each other, staying at each other's homes when they visit. Reminiscent of other intentionally formed families outside of traditional routes, such as the extended gay and lesbian families Kath Weston (1997) writes about, Louis characterized their relationship with that set of IPs as "friendship that's grown into a family." Many women indicated that they desired a similar relationship with their IPs, though only these two families in my study reported achieving it. Instead, for many there was an intense connection between surrogates' families and IPs during the journey, followed by a decrease in contact after the birth.

This shift in familial relations was concerning to many women, especially those who had been on multiple journeys and had already experienced it. Because of this, some surrogates were hesitant about allowing their children to form close relationships with IPs. This was especially common among surrogates with young children, who were more likely to express concern about their children being unable to understand the sudden loss of contact with IPs. While all of the surrogates in my study indicated that they introduced their children to at least one set of their IPs, some, especially experienced surrogates, were more cautious with early or extended contact.

For example, Dawn Rudge, a one-time surrogate who had birthed twins and was the mother of three young children, decided to wait to introduce her children to her IPs until the pregnancy had established itself. I asked her to explain, and we had the following exchange:

> DAWN: The transfer was in November. We waited until March before I let [my children] meet [the IPs]. Because I wanted to make sure that we got to a gestation where they were probably going to stay and we didn't have to worry about a loss. So they met them in March.
>
> HEATHER: Why was that important for you, to wait for your kids to meet them until March?
>
> DAWN: I just felt like if [the IPs] backed out or if we did lose [the twins] and [the IPs] were not able to emotionally handle it, that it would be more devastating to my kids to have them meet somebody—bring them into their lives and then they go away—than just to wait until everything was okay and everybody was good, and we knew that this was probably going to be a sure thing. I'm not sure exactly why, other than I just wanted to really protect my kids and not get them involved in something until I knew that it was all going to work out well.

Once the pregnancy was established and Dawn knew that her IPs were "going to stay," she introduced her children to them. They met only a couple other times though, "maybe two or three," Dawn said, once "at one of the sonogram appointments with the perinatologist and then one of the normal doctor's visits." Her IM, Sharon, also accompanied Dawn on a field trip with her older daughter's school class. Dawn was thirty weeks pregnant at the time, and she was "just a little uncomfortable" being on the trip "if something was to go wrong." So she asked Sharon to join them. During that trip, Ivy, her daughter, and Sharon "got to bond."

Like many of the surrogates in my study, for Dawn the establishment of a connection between the IPs and her children was important. This was not so much because surrogates wanted their children to develop relationships with the IPs, but because they wanted their children to have a good understanding of why they were surrogates and where the surro-babies were going after birth. Dawn put it this way: "So I think it was good because they knew Sharon and Gary. They had spent a little bit of time with them, more Sharon than Gary. So they knew where the babies were going." Other surrogates also deliberately structured interactions between their children and IPs to ensure that their children understood the surrogacy arrangement and the fate of the babies. In doing so, however, many women were cautious about putting their children in situations where they could potentially become invested in relationships with IPs and then have their feelings hurt if IPs reduced or cut off contact.

According to the women in my study, children sometimes do get hurt in their relationships with IPs. This occurred for Ann Beltran's youngest two children. Ann's first IPs lived several states away, and therefore, her four children did not develop close relationships with them. When the IPs came to visit, "they were really great with the kids," Ann told me, "but that was it. It wasn't constantly trying to bring them into everything. So there was a real line." Ann's second set of IPs, however, lived nearby and tried to establish close relationships with the entire Beltran family. According to Ann, during the surrogacy journey, the new IPs, Donny and Phyllis, "were always inviting and trying to do things with our children all the time." Ann was initially hesitant about the level of involvement her IPs desired, but her husband convinced her to do as they wanted, saying, "Oh, Donny's great, and they're just very open, loving people."

The two families became close and participated together in many social events, with the children involved. Before the birth of the babies, "we would go down and visit [Donny and Phyllis] all the time," Ann said, "and they invited us down, and they really wanted to be part of our family." The families spent a lot of time together, and her children came to "love Donny and Phyllis, and Donny and Phyllis wanted that type of relationship is what they had said."

Donny and Phyllis pushed familial-like relationships with Ann's children and made explicit promises to them about continued contact after the surro-twins were born. Phyllis, for example, had said "all this stuff" to Ann's younger daughter, "like, 'Oh Madelyn, you're going to be able to take care of [the babies].'

And all this kind of stuff." According to Ann, Madelyn was very excited about the arrival of the babies and greatly anticipated caring for them. "My little Madelyn," Ann said, "is probably the biggest little mama in the world. She's very kind of nurturing and loves little kids."

Things changed, however, once the surro-twins were born. Just before the birth Donny and Phyllis decided they did not want Madelyn or her younger brother (Ann's youngest two children) around their family until the babies were at least three months old, which they then extended to a six-month delay. Ann was devastated for her children. She explained:

> All of a sudden, last minute before the twins were born, they [Donny and Phyllis] decided that they didn't want the children to see the twins. And it was because they thought, "Well, we don't want them carrying any germs to the hospital." And that was probably the hardest part because my two oldest got to see them, but then the two youngest, who really like Donny and Phyllis, the IPs, were just kind of devastated. Because they came to see me [in the hospital] and they wanted to see Phyllis and Donny and the twins and—so that really broke my heart, I think, just that they would, at the last minute, decide to do that. So I definitely feel bad about that part.

Ann found this so problematic that she now wishes she had not allowed her children to have developed such close ties to the IPs. She confessed: "I don't think I would have done that again or chosen that road. I would have had much more distance, I think." Ann went so far as to tell me that knowing what she now does, she wishes she had not chosen to work with Donny and Phyllis. Despite this, Ann saw positive benefits deriving from the overall surrogacy experience for her children, which was typical of the other women in my study.

CHILD BENEFITS

Surrogates did not enter into surrogacy with the goal of helping their children to grow emotionally. Instead, most women were concerned about how surrogacy could negatively affect their children. As Molly Hughes told me, "I never went into it thinking what they would get out of it, really. I just knew I didn't want them to be traumatized by it or anything!" However, surrogates retrospectively identified surrogacy as a "good learning experience" for their children. Molly and the other women in my study told me that their children learned important life lessons from surrogacy. "I think in a roundabout way they learn that life isn't the same for everybody." Molly continued. "They know some people want babies and can't have them." According to April Palmer, surrogacy was a "good lesson for our whole family." Many women indicated that the lessons learned from surrogacy were unique or more challenging to teach children in what they characterized as today's "instant gratification" and "self-indulgent" culture. April explained:

> It was great for my kids to grow up witnessing that life isn't about taking, but sometimes about giving. I don't know that in today's society that we stress that very much with kids. [With] a lot of parents the kids get whatever they want, and we want to keep kids happy or whatever. So any time I have an opportunity to teach my kids lessons about "it's not all about you," I try to do that. So that was probably a good life experience for them, as a parent [for me] to give to my children—that you can be selfless. There can be things you do in life that are sacrifices [you make] for other people.

The other women in my study also hoped their children would come to appreciate the value of self-sacrifice and altruism. Some women noted that they were beginning to see this lesson bear fruit in their children's daily lives. Rhonda Chapman, for example, told me that following her surrogacy journey she noticed that her son was more considerate toward others. She gave me the example of their weekly trip to a popular family restaurant that has games. While her family was adept at winning the "claw machine" and getting four or five stuffed animals on each visit, other children were not. Her son was soon approaching other children and handing out his "extra animals" to them. Rhonda was pleased and attributed this to "learning by [her] example." Her son learned "that we had one [child] and we were happy, and we wanted someone else to be happy too." She said: "We never had to push him to give [the stuffed animals] up. He always wanted to. I mean he wanted to have one for himself, but he always wanted to make another child happy. We would have a people come up to us just to say, 'You should be really proud of your son.' So yeah, I think [surrogacy] was a good thing for him." Rhonda was pleased that her son learned to share with others and to have a "giving heart." Learning to sacrifice was one of the important positive benefits for their children that many women identified.

Surrogacy was viewed by my participants as an activity that affected both individual members and the family as a whole. Participating in surrogacy was seen as a team effort that could have rewards for both individuals and the family, including learning important life lessons and becoming "better people." Families have to adapt to the demands of surrogacy work: husbands abstain from sex with their wives, children sacrifice family trips to the water park so that mom can rest, and daughters traipse into rest area bathrooms to inject their mothers with Lupron. Surrogates expressed guilt over the sacrifices their families made so that they could participate in surrogacy as well as hope that important life lessons emerge. As Molly Hughes said about the impact of surrogacy on her children, "I think they're learning . . . that you've got to make sacrifices. They're making sacrifices, and it doesn't have anything to do with them, it doesn't have anything to do with me. It has to do with these people they've never met. But they know that we're all coming together to try [to] do this incredible thing for someone. I don't know that they can fully realize the impact of it yet, but I think that they will someday be able to look back and say, 'Wow! My mom did something amazing for someone else.'"

Conclusion

A recent *New York Times* article on surrogacy law referred to surrogacy arrangements as a way for women "to stay home and raise their own children" (Lewin 2014). While surrogacy may temporarily allow women who previously worked to avoid outside paid employment, given the amount of labor surrogates engage in, the idea that surrogacy is primarily home-based work conducive to full-time (self-sufficient) mothering seems a simplistic reading of these arrangements. I see that reading as based on several basic misconceptions about surrogacy. The first, which might come from an unfamiliarity with the world of IVF via third-party reproduction, is that surrogacy equates to regular pregnancy (and that regular pregnancy is not work). The temporal and physical demands of commercial surrogacy in the United States on surrogates are different from those present in a pregnancy obtained for oneself (using one's own body and gametes) without the assistance of reproductive technologies. The monitoring needed to sustain the pregnancy, the labor needed to coordinate the medical protocol, and the social demands of third-party pregnancy are also distinctly different from anything involved in a "regular" pregnancy. There are similarities, of course, between surrogacy and nonsurrogacy pregnancies, but the additional labor load of surrogacy cannot easily be pushed behind the door of stay-at-home mothering.

My research reveals that instead surrogacy creates family work, a kind of third shift for reproductive workers and their families, similar to the way the demands of home create a second shift for contemporary workers following their first shift of paid labor (Hochschild 1989). Family work is not the paid labor of women's day jobs and not the home and family obligations of the second shift. In fact, family work—the labor of third-party reproduction—is not quite work or family, but a liminal state in between. It is not the time-card-punching labor of paid work, which was viewed by many in my study as necessary but unfulfilling. Nor does it neatly map onto the experiences of women who conceive, gestate, and bear children of their own outside the reproductive marketplace. Rather, for the surrogate—and often for her husband and sometimes for her children as well—the experience of surrogacy becomes part hobby, part job, part sociability, and part domestic work. It is woven into the fabric of the day-to-day lived experience of these women and their families. Everyone participates in this cottage industry of baby making, but not without tension.

The women in my study articulated the conflicts they experienced between the second shift of home and family and what I am conceptualizing as a third shift of family work. This tension is ironic in that the rules of surrogacy require women to be mothers, yet the surrogacy industry is organized in ways that are somewhat unfriendly to today's complicated families. As I have explored in this chapter, surrogacy-related work activities do not always accommodate young children or the complicated home lives of working parents and socially active children. Surrogates are therefore expected to have supportive adult family members available to assist them through their surrogacies. The organization of commercial surrogacy relies on those other workers in the family—husbands, partners, and older children—who can absorb the extra labor inherent in and a consequence of reproductive work. Surrogates are expected to be both involved, caring mothers (which in the market is an indicator that a candidate is suitable for surrogacy) and women who are able to easily extract themselves from family responsibilities—at least temporarily—to engage in surrogacy activities. Like other forms of care work, my research reveals a picture, therefore, of surrogates laboring to make families for others while that labor often takes them away from their own (for the similar impact of child-care work on workers, see Hondagneu-Sotelo 2001; MacDonald 2010; Parrenas 2001).

For many women, the consequence of that tension between the second shift of home and the third shift of the family work of surrogacy was guilt. Most women indicated that participating in surrogacy involved some level of guilt for them. Because of the way domestic tasks in the home were gendered for most women, surrogates spoke of feeling a gap between what they wanted to or could provide—or usually did provide—for their families and what they were able to do, once they added the demands of surrogacy to their already busy schedules. They understood that care gap as temporary, and almost everyone in my study argued that it was only a momentary inconvenience that they and their families willingly endured to help their IPs bring their children into the world. Yet they found that tension problematic at times, and laced with guilt. This guilt was only exacerbated when relations with IPs soured, when embryo transfers were continually unsuccessful, or when surrogates felt their IPs did not adequately appreciate their familial sacrifices.

The surrogacy industry attempts to make accommodations for that care gap (and that guilt) by including in surrogates' contracts reimbursements for child care and housecleaning (paid for by IPs). Some women in my study took advantage of those contractual obligations and hired babysitters and housecleaners when needed. However, as shown in this chapter, I found that other women were reluctant to take advantage of those funds, due to preferences for family-based care and housework and the desire to be prudent with IPs' money. This is reminiscent of the ways some paid employees are reluctant to use family-friendly benefits (such as maternity leave or flextime) even though doing so would assist

them (Hochschild 1997). Hiring others to perform labor did not fix the problem
entirely, because for many women the issue is guilt about not being able to provide that labor themselves. This was the case with surrogates. It was not simply
that they wanted the work to get done, the children to be transported, or the Six
Flags trip to occur, but that they wanted to complete those tasks or participate
in those events themselves. At its core, I see this as mother guilt, the guilt felt by
many contemporary women about not being able to do it all (Hays 1996).

The guilt of mothers about the choices they make and how they understand
them to affect their children is not unique to surrogacy. In fact, many scholars
point to it as a normal aspect of the cultural construction of contemporary
motherhood, especially in the middle class. Mothers today engage in—or feel
pressured to engage in—what Sharon Hays has called "intensive mothering"
(1996, 4), Annette Lareau calls "concerted cultivation" (2003, 2), and Margaret
Nelson terms "parenting out of control" (2010). These concepts articulate a
historically constructed ideology centered on an intensive hovering of mothers
over their children; a focus on the minutiae of children's lives rather than on
the mothers who care for them; an investment, day in and day out, of women's
lives (and their time and money) in children; and the privileging of children's
perceived needs over those of their mothers. Intensive mothering is explicitly
gendered, with ideas about good mothering explicitly linked to the degree to
which women devote their time, money, and energy to, and focus their lives on,
their children (Hays 1996). Ironically, at the same time, the majority of mothers
with children in the United States work outside of the home. According to the
Bureau of Labor Statistics (2014), the labor force participation rate for women
with children under the age of eighteen was 69.9 percent. Even for those with
children under the age of six, the participation rate was 63.9 percent. This combination of the high percentage of working mothers and the ideology of intensive mothering creates a complicated terrain for women. As Hays has argued,
"modern-day mothers are facing two socially constructed cultural images of
what a good mother looks like"—the "traditional" stay-at-home mother who is
intensely focused on her children and the "supermom" who can be seen "effort-
lessly juggling home and work" (1996, 131–33). Because of this, Hays continues,
women face a "cultural ambivalence," creating a "no-win situation" when it
comes to decisions about work and family. At a time that is characterized by
intensive mothering, increased numbers of women in the workforce, and changing gender relations in the home and workplace, the choices women make about
work and family are, therefore, often infused with guilt.

What is interesting about surrogacy and mother guilt is the way that the
dominant framing of surrogacy in the United States, which resists conceptualizations of surrogacy as work, influences the guilt women feel about their surrogacy labor. Surrogates' guilt does not precisely match the typical guilt of the
contemporary working mother. Surrogates do not feel guilty because they have

to go to work (as surrogates) but because the care they are giving to the families of others sometimes keeps them for caring for their own. Most surrogates indicated that they felt guilty about the sacrifices their children and husbands made so that they could be surrogates. They felt guilty about the extra work their husbands and older children took on during surrogacies, and the time they themselves had to spend away from home for surrogacy-related appointments. They felt guilty when they could not participate in family activities because of an appointment with the RE, or when their children missed them because they were on post-transfer bed rest and could not have visitors.

That guilt was particularly acute because, as my research reveals, surrogates understand surrogacy to be an enjoyable pursuit—not work—that they engage in out of their love of pregnancy and desire to help others. Surrogacy work is not work they do on behalf of their families to feed and clothe their children, which are often reasons mothers give to help assuage the guilt they feel because of their paid labor (Damaske 2011). In the world of surrogacy in the United States, financial need is not culturally appropriate as a justification for surrogacy work. Rather, women told me that they engaged in surrogacy because they want to do so, because they enjoy it, not because they need to do it for their families.

Like the majority of American mothers, most of the women in my study were employed in paid work outside of the home, and most felt some guilt about the choices they made about their careers and caring for their children. My participants reported that they thought of surrogacy as quite distinct from their regular day jobs. Surrogacy is not a job, they insisted, but a calling, a sacrifice, a hobby, a gift—and one that they intensely enjoy. It is precisely because of the intense enjoyment they experience that they feel so much guilt about what they see as the familial sacrifices their children and husbands make in order for them to be surrogates. Many told me that surrogacy is a selfish pursuit and that this is why they felt so much guilt. According to the ideology of intensive mothering, today good mothers focus on their children and their children's happiness—not their own. Surrogates parlay their guilt, therefore, into decisions they make about compensation.

Surrogacy in the United States in the first two decades of the twenty-first century is family work, with everyone pitching in and everyone seemingly positioned to reap the rewards of character development and compensation. The structure and rhetoric of surrogacy, its reliance on family support, and the expected involvement of surrogates' family members in various aspects of the surrogacy journey all facilitate a framing of surrogacy as family sacrifice, rather than employment, thus helping obscure surrogacy as paid labor and surrogates as workers.

CHAPTER 6

Obscured Labor

As I began to write this chapter, news broke that the first birth resulting from a uterine transplant had occurred. Swedish doctors reported in the *Lancet* (Brännström et al. 2015) that they had successfully transplanted a uterus from a sixty-one-year-old woman into one of their patients, a thirty-five-year-old woman born without a uterus but with functioning ovaries. Their patient underwent in vitro fertilization (IVF) using her own eggs one year after the transplant and gave birth in September 2014 to a healthy son. The media reported that two more uterine transplant births were expected to occur within the next several weeks (Associated Press 2014; "Baby Is Born to Woman Who Received Womb Transplant" 2014).

This medical breakthrough made me wonder if surrogacy was eventually going to become obsolete. Would intended mothers (IMs) want to receive uterine transplants instead of using surrogates? Given the invasive medical procedure involved, the expense, and how new the procedure is, perhaps not—but what about ten or fifteen years in the future, especially if there are high success rates? Based on my interviews with intended parents (IPs), it would not be out of line to presume that many would at least seriously consider the option. IPs invest considerable time and expense in their quest for children. And several IMs told me that they would jump at the chance to give birth themselves if only they could get their hands on a working uterus. Uterine transplants, of course, would not assist those women who have conditions contraindicative or posing significant challenges to pregnancy (such as lupus) or those for whom their inability to carry a pregnancy or birth a live child was attributed to nonuterine issues. But for those with "absolute uterine infertility, which is caused by absence of the uterus or the presence of a nonfunctional uterus," uterine transplant offers "the first available treatment" (Brännström et al. 2015, 607).

The first uterine transplant birth also made me wonder if transplants could perform all the roles of surrogacy. The ultimate goal of surrogacy is the birth of live babies for those who cannot (or will not) birth children themselves. Everyone in surrogacy is united on this goal: the IPs, the medical practitioners, the surrogacy agencies, and the surrogates. However, as I have explored in various chapters in this book, for surrogates surrogacy in and of itself has become a goal, a motivator, and a desired experience. My research reveals that women largely participate in surrogacy for what they gain from it (which is not a baby): the pleasure of pregnancy, the fulfillment of helping others, the relationships cultivated with IPs, and, yes, the money.

Research on surrogacy over the course of the past thirty years, especially the psychological literature, has revealed that the altruistic pull to help others and the enjoyment of pregnancy have always been central to women's stated motivations for participating in surrogacy (see, for example, Berend 2012; Ciccarelli and Beckman 2005; Edelmann 2004; Field 1990; Hanafin 1984; Ragone 1994 and 1999; van den Akker 2007). While most surrogates in the past at least had the option of compensation (even if they did not take it), and while there are still women who engage in altruistic surrogacy (that is, unpaid surrogacy), in the United States today the default is compensated surrogacy.

There has been tremendous growth in the surrogacy market and in the revenue generated, both for the industry and for individual women. Surrogacy has become part of a hugely profitable reproductive-industrial complex in the United States, unregulated by the federal government and by most states. This industry, which as a whole is estimated to generate $3 billion annually, has recruited many women to participate as surrogates, many of whom have repeat journeys (Spar 2006, 3). As shown in earlier chapters, the medical practice has also changed quite dramatically since the 1980s. The procedure of artificial insemination in traditional surrogacy was much simpler than the intense and invasive medical protocol of IVF involved in gestational surrogacy today. With the expansion of the surrogacy market and the medical advances of IVF surrogacy, there are more journeys overall, with more women in total working as surrogates—and on average they each have more journeys. Working as a surrogate today is also more labor intensive than it was in past decades, due to the complex medical protocol and the propensity of women to engage in repeat journeys.

In this book I have examined surrogacy as work. This is a particular framing of surrogacy. According to William Gamson and Gadi Wolfsfeld, a frame is a "central organizing idea, suggesting what is at issue. It deals with the pattern-organizing aspect of meaning" (1993, 118). Other scholars have used different frames to examine surrogacy. For example, Susan Markens uses a social constructionist frame in *Surrogate Motherhood and the Politics of Reproduction* (2007) to analyze the legislative debates in New York and California on the subject. Much of the academic literature on surrogacy uses a psychological problems frame, focusing on analyzing the psychological character of surrogates and attempting to determine a unique psychological profile for this group of women that would explain their participation in surrogacy (see, for example, Anleu 1992; Ciccarelli and Beckman 2005; Edelmann 2004; Field 1990; Hanafin 1984; Ketchum 1992; Oliver 1989; Purdy 1996; van den Akker 2007). A stratification frame is used in much of the feminist literature to argue that surrogacy practices both strengthen and produce inequality (Corea 1985; D. Roberts 1997; Rothman 1989).

As I mentioned at the beginning of this book, I became interested in exploring surrogacy through the frame of work once I began talking with surrogates and learned of the tremendous amount of labor in which they are engaged. I am not unique in thinking about surrogacy as work. In fact, thinking about surrogacy this way is a framing commonly used by those opposed to surrogacy. As I explored in earlier chapters, using the work framing to argue against surrogacy is two-pronged. The first prong positions surrogacy as the commodification of women's bodies and the exploitation of poor women in the reproductive baby market. This framing is common in much of the feminist literature focused on stratification, both in the research that arose following the Baby M case and the more recent literature examining the globalized surrogacy market. The second prong, which positions surrogates as "money-hungry uterine whores" who pimp their uteruses to the highest bidder, can be seen in much of the popular media accounts of surrogacy and the online discourse surrounding those stories (such as in the comments section in online editions of newspapers). Both prongs, which problematize surrogates as workers, have been prevalent in the decades-old debate about surrogacy that has waxed and waned in the United States since the early days of the industry in the 1980s.

My examination of surrogacy as work differs from the anti-surrogacy framing in that it is not meant as a condemnation of these practices but rather presents an empirically based examination of surrogacy from multiple perspectives (those of surrogates, IPs, surrogacy professionals, and surrogates' family members), showing that surrogacy is not simple exploitation. My interest in framing surrogacy as work began with my initial interest in the amount of labor in which women engage to birth children for others—many of whom they did not know at the beginning of their journeys—and the intensity with which that work is obscured through the structure of the industry, market practices, and individuals in the community. Through the chapters in this book I have pursued a more nuanced examination of contemporary practices based on the ethnographic data I collected. The beginning of this book opened with the questions of why surrogacy work is hidden labor and why there is such strong resistance to thinking about and talking about the labor of surrogates. Through the chapters that followed, I have provided and explored empirical evidence of that resistance in various contexts, on the part of the contemporary surrogacy marketplace, agencies, surrogates' families, and surrogates, as well as in surrogates' relationships with IPs. I conclude this book by returning to those original questions. Through an examination of the various meanings compensation holds for surrogates, how money operates for women, and how various players deal with the work framings that are inherent in receiving compensation for expended effort, in this chapter I directly confront the question of obscured labor and contemplate what it has to say about the larger relationship among women, the children they bear, and the reproductive marketplace.

MONEY RULES

A good place to confront the obscuring of surrogate labor is to examine surrogates' relationships to the compensation they receive. As discussed earlier in this book, first-time surrogates generally make between $15,000 and $25,000, and experienced surrogates between $20,000 and $35,000, per surrogacy journey. This amount represents a portion of the fees paid by IPs for surrogacy. The bulk of IPs' costs are for medical expenses (which typically run $20,000–$30,000 per IVF cycle, with many IPs needing more than one cycle to achieve pregnancy).

Money for service is emblematic of paid employment. As I have explored throughout this book, positioning surrogates as workers is a problematic position culturally and socially in the United States. Because of this, there are elaborate rules and rituals regarding the money surrogates receive. I think of these as money rules, which surrogates are socialized to follow. Money rules determine how money is discussed, when it is paid, when and with whom to talk about it, appropriate feelings to have toward it, and correct framings of its meaning. Some of these rules are explicit in agency guidelines; others are implied in surrogates' interactions with other surrogates and surrogacy professionals. Together, these explicit and implicit rules help create a particular culture of norms about behavior and speech regarding money in the surrogacy community in the United States. These money rules are essential to the obscuring of surrogate labor.

It is important to note that these money rules are cultural rules, not legal ones. As discussed earlier in this book, as of this writing, twenty-nine states have statutes or case law regarding surrogacy, and most of those are supportive of the practice. In the remaining twenty-one states, the legality of surrogacy has not been tested. Only one state, New York, and the District of Columbia have imposed criminal penalties for compensated surrogacy. Therefore, money rules by and large deal with cultural edicts against surrogacy, not legal ones.

Money rules are visible from the beginning of a surrogacy journey and can be seen in the initial screening process of surrogates. As discussed in earlier chapters, agencies evaluate the initial motivations of individual surrogates in an attempt to protect themselves and the industry from scrutiny and criticism. Women in financial straits and women on welfare are (usually) disqualified by agencies. Likewise, women who make it known that they are attempting to make a quick buck are not welcome in most established agencies. Selecting women who display a proper orientation to surrogacy—one not focused on money, but on altruistic giving and a love of pregnancy—is an important strategy employed by surrogacy agencies and those lawyers and reproductive endocrinologists (REs) who broker matches between IPs and surrogates. For surrogacy to function properly, money cannot be the explicitly stated primary goal, I was told over and over again in my interviews with agency owners and workers, surrogates, and their family members.

This money rule was often framed as a way to protect surrogates from the experience of surrogacy. This can be seen in the comments of Deidre Richards, herself a surrogate and owner of a small surrogacy agency, when she was explaining what she looks for in a surrogate: "The desire for being a surrogate and carrying someone else's child has to be first and foremost. I know the money is nice for a lot of them, but it can't be their main goal. Because if it is, they're not going to be happy throughout the journey, because there's so much more involved in it than just getting a paycheck every month." Focusing on money "only leads to [the surrogate's] disappointment," Deidre concluded. Surrogates themselves were quite vocal on this point in their interviews with me. In fact, many women argued that both their motives for pursuing surrogacy and their experiences as surrogates were so disparate from the compensation that their fees were not—and should not be considered—commensurate pay for their work. The comments of Tina Vargas were indicative of this perspective. Tina told me that surrogacy "is just not all about money, because it isn't enough for what you have to go through." She continued:

> I mean, there's people who have triplets and people who—I mean, there are some horror stories of things that people have to go through, like collapsed lungs and having to go through surgeries. And being pregnant and that's it. They won't be able to be surrogates again because of these physical things. But [there are] so many other things that could go wrong during the pregnancy. There's no way that money is going to make up for that time that you've lost, even just being on bed rest. And time lost in the hospital if you have these major surgeries or things that come up—being sick. So there's no way I could ever agree that it's about the money, because it's just not.

Money rules encourage women to adhere to a particular way of thinking about surrogacy and talking about their motivations. These rules explicitly focus on women's feelings and, most importantly, the expression of those feelings. Women need to have their feelings properly aligned, I was told, to successfully complete their surrogacy journeys and to ensure that they feel good about themselves. They must engage in what Arlie Hochschild calls "emotional labor" (1983, 7)— an aligning of one's emotions for the purpose of the market—for surrogacy to function properly. Surrogates should feel an altruistic impulse toward helping others and a physical delight in the pregnant state, this money rule dictates, but they should not—or should not primarily—feel a desire for money; they should especially not feel a desire for more money, nor should they think about surrogacy as a permanent job opportunity. Surrogates told me that thinking about surrogacy as work or a job, and depending on compensation for it as one does a paycheck puts one in a dangerous position emotionally, financially, and socially. It also poses a threat to the cultural palatability of surrogacy and, therefore, the industry, and the surrogacy community discourages it through the use of money rules.

The negative discourse surrounding women's participation in reproductive work for money was so strongly felt by my participants that even talking about the money was uncomfortable for many of them. Many women discussed with me the negative portrayal of surrogates in the media and their desire to "right that wrong." Recall the comments of Rosalyn Whelan when she told me "most surrogates—if you call [surrogacy] a job, they just get very, very angry, very upset." Discussions of money are so closely linked to antisurrogacy discourse in the popular media and general public that talking about compensation was occasionally a challenge in my interviews with surrogates. Several women were reluctant to even discuss it. One of the counselors I interviewed, Martha Griffin, who has worked in the field of reproduction for decades, contextualized this reluctance for me when she noted that among her clients there was a feeling of shame attached to being a surrogate. Surrogacy for pay is often negatively characterized, Martha reported, as a desperate act of desperate women. "And that has shame attached to it," Martha went on:

> Because I've had people say [to surrogates I counsel], "Well, if you need money that badly, we'll make you a loan." So it's like as if—now if they were selling Avon, no one would say that to them. But when people hear that they're doing it for money, it seems like they're very desperate. It's like stripping after the kids go to bed or something. They feel like there's something desperate about doing this for money. So I've had surrogates sort of be taken aback how people perceive that they must *only* be doing it because they really need the money.

Due to these negative characterizations of women who work as surrogates, many seek to minimize the role compensation plays in their motivations to pursue surrogacy work. By and large, this "feeling rule"—what Hochschild identifies as "the emotive requirements situations call forth" (1979, 572)—is effective: all of the women in my study but one adhered to this rule, at least in what they said to me. They told me that they wanted to be surrogates because they loved being pregnant, they wanted to help others, and they enjoyed the relationships they developed with their IPs. Their feelings seemingly followed the socially appropriate expression of surrogate motivation and desire. The surrogacy market requires this emotional labor, the work that must be done to cope with "feeling rules", and creates mechanisms for its management. Surrogates undergo a socialization process in which they "learned what surrogacy was really about" and realized the negative characterizations that accompany publicly speaking of engaging in surrogacy to make money. Surrogacy is fun, they told me, it is a sacrifice, but it is not a very good moneymaker (even if that was what originally brought one to the idea of surrogacy). Through the socialization process that occurs in interactions with surrogacy professionals and other surrogates, the women in my study came to understand that to make sense of what they put their bodies through and to protect themselves from disappointment, they have to receive additional benefits beyond compensation from surrogacy; and all of my study participants told me that they did receive such benefits.

Some of the women, however, pushed back against this money rule. Two participants spoke quite freely with me about their original desire for compensation. While one of them went on to tell me that she now understood the importance of engaging in surrogacy "for the right reasons," the other, Allison Farro, unapologetically continued to discuss her interest in compensation. She told me: "Honestly, it [the idea of being a surrogate] started out as the money would be nice and I'd be doing something good. But probably the biggest motivator was the money." Allison went on to describe having an "excellent journey" and continuing relationship with her IPs. She also told me that she was looking into working for another agency because of their increased compensation packages. Other women insisted that while they considered their own motivations to be altruistic, they see nothing wrong in others, like Allison, engaging in surrogacy primarily for the monetary benefits.

Overall, however, surrogates often talk about "the heart"—not money—in discussing their work. This was true when Helena Ragone (1994) studied traditional surrogates in the 1980s, and it remains true today. In my interviews with them, surrogates equated "the heart" with altruistic motivations and loving kindness and "the head" with economic motivations and calculations. Some women used a heart-head dichotomy when they explained the proper way to think about surrogacy. They told me that surrogates need to approach surrogacy with their hearts, not primarily with their heads. Only people who feel surrogacy with their hearts can truly comprehend it. Using one's head to approach surrogacy and thinking about it as a moneymaker indicated that one did not understand surrogacy, I was told. For example, when Rosalyn Whelan discussed being confronted in public by people who asked her how much money she made as a surrogate, she said those questions showed that the people who asked them "cannot truly understand surrogacy." She continued: "If your heart is really not in that place and you have to think with your head, then the first thing that comes to your mind is money. So it is kind of hard to convince someone who doesn't really feel it, who doesn't understand it, that it is about emotions, it is about helping somebody. It's not about money. They just don't believe you. They just don't get it."

Agencies and the surrogacy community encourage women to observe this rule. In fact, I would argue that the agencies and the surrogacy community almost create a script for women to follow—what Kieran Healy in his work on blood and organ donation calls "contexts for giving" that "elicit altruistic action" (2006, 67). If women want to become surrogates, for whatever reason, they must adhere to the "organizational mechanisms that provide people with reasons and opportunities" to do so (ibid., 2). The organizational context of surrogacy and the cultural norms regarding reproduction produce a neat script for altruism, which people involved then insist on. Those women who refuse to follow the script and the money rules and who make it known that they are primarily interested in surrogacy because of the compensation are simply usually not hired by agencies. They can attempt to make independent arrangements (making their own matches with IPs outside of agencies)—and some do, I was told—but they must then be vetted by IPs and REs, many of whom do adhere to the money rules.

This is not to argue that women wanting to become surrogates do not have altruistic motivations prior to their socialization within the industry. Only several of my participants did not report having altruistic impulses from the beginning of their interest in surrogacy. Of course, they were reporting those motivations retrospectively, after they had participated in surrogacy and in the socialization process. However, they also reported other, even stronger interests—their desire to be pregnant again and, in some cases, their need to supplement their household income. Those interests are acknowledged by the industry and are also a part of the surrogate motivational script. However, the money rules dominate, especially in surrogates' interactions with organizations and people who may be anti surrogacy.

As women move through the surrogacy market, they become socialized to follow those particular norms and the script, and they then work to socialize others to share their belief of what surrogacy is really about. Many women reported interactions with strangers in public as opportunities to educate others about surrogacy. Participants in my study were especially vocal about this when recalling questions by strangers in public about compensation. Women would work to minimize their overall compensation figure, for example by replying to questions about how much they make as surrogates with comments such as "about as much as you can make from a part-time job."

As I explored above, surrogates also police themselves and socialize women with "proper motivations" into the community. For example, Leah Spalding— who said that she was initially interested in surrogacy because of the money she could earn—told me about being approached by others with similar orientations to surrogacy: "Mostly the people who have asked me about it are financially

driven. They want the money. I've never once met a person—except for the support group [of other surrogates in my agency], obviously—never met somebody
who wants to do this just because they are helping someone, or because they
value family and they believe that everyone should have what some people can't
have, you know? Mostly people will say—one person e-mailed and said, "Oh,
you know, how did you get into that? How much do they pay you?" When Leah
received such inquiries, she steered people toward the proper way of thinking
about surrogacy:

> Before I give them any information about the agency, I say, "Why do you want
> to get into it?" Kind of puts them on the spot. And some of them say, "Well,
> honestly, I want the money." And others are trying, "Well, I don't really know.
> I've heard you get a lot of money. It might be really fun." So, it's like, "Be hon-
> est. Tell me you want the money because I used to be you, searching the [Inter]
> net, how can I make some easy money?" And it took that time for me to learn.
> So, those people—well, the one that said, "Well, honestly, I just want the
> money." I said, "Well, you know what? I really don't suggest you do it because
> not only is this really stressful and hard on your body and you have to deal
> with a lot of things, this is something that you should want to do because you
> want to help someone or because you value certain things. Not because of the
> money."

Many of the interactions that surrogates have in public with women who
are contemplating surrogacy follow the money rules. Leah's responses affirm
nonmarket framings of surrogacy, protecting surrogacy from criticism, and
aim to align potential surrogates with the proper way to approach one's stated
motivations.

Despite the socialization efforts of women like Leah and the screening procedures agencies use, all of the agency directors with whom I spoke let me know
that there were women in their programs whom they had hired and whom they
then later suspected of being primarily motivated by money. Surrogates also
reported that they were aware of other women primarily motivated by money
who worked as surrogates. These women "let their true colors show," I was told,
once they were matched and in surrogacy arrangements with IPs. They are
"easy to spot," according to Martha Griffin. She also told me that women who
are primarily motivated by money sometimes do not even acknowledge that
to themselves. She intimated that what I am calling the money rules were so
strongly felt that some women were hesitant to admit even to themselves their
interest in compensation. Others are apparently bolder in their disregard of
the money rules. Sherry Woods, for example, told me that some women "just
pretend" to be correctly motivated: "People treat us like we're money-grubbing
uterine whores. Well, you know what? Some of them are! But they try to pretend
they're not."

Surrogates—and surrogacy professionals—distanced themselves from such women. Notice how Sherry attempted to do this by moving from the first person plural ("us") to the third person plural ("them") when referring to "money-grubbing uterine whores." This can also be seen in the comments of Laurel Molza: "There are a lot of ladies out there that will do it strictly [for money]; because they'll do pregnancy back to back to back. And you know that they're in it for the fee, which is fine. If that's their motivation and that's what they want to do, far be it from me to say anything. That's just not my motivation and why I wanted to be a surrogate." Most surrogates who indicated that they knew such women problematized them, characterizing their journeys as difficult ones because those women were too focused on money, losing sight of what the women in my study called the "real meaning of surrogacy."

Being money hungry not only has the potential to make surrogacy look bad in the eyes of others, but it was also seen to be indicative of more serious character flaws. Money-hungry surrogates—those who can be used as examples of women who rent their wombs—are therefore used as cautionary tales to guide agencies in the proper selection of surrogates. They are also used as justification for restricting the number of times women can engage in surrogacy. Professionals reported concerns about women becoming addicted to surrogacy, especially to the money they can make as surrogates. Because of this, many agencies try to restrict their surrogates to three journeys (though two women in my sample had completed more than three). There are a number of factors that come into play in limiting the number of journeys, especially the recommendations of medical professionals who warn of the increase in potential negative health incidents related to bearing multiple children. But this rule of limiting the number of journeys is also about monitoring women's motivations and attempting to ensure that none are misdirected. This can be seen in the comments of Janice Holberg, an agency director who limits her surrogates to three journeys. Janice explained that she prefers women to limit themselves to two journeys and will "take them a third time, but we don't really like for them to do it more than that because then you have to start questioning their motivation." When I asked Janice, "What in particular would you be concerned about?" she replied: "Why they're wanting to be pregnant that much. Or have they become addicted to the money so to speak, or something like that? So we always have a little concern for those who want to do it more than three times." Other surrogacy professionals told me they found something problematic about these women, as they can be viewed as professional surrogates, women for whom surrogacy has become employment and who can be used as fodder for criticism against the industry.

Ironically, however, at the same time that agencies actively limit the number of surrogates' journeys, they rely on experienced surrogates and the skills they have gained through their surrogacy work. Cindy Woltz, for example, was "pulled out of retirement" for her fifth journey when her agency had a set of IPs who seemed to be particularly difficult. The agency wanted "a special woman" who would be able to deal with the IPs as their surrogate. Cindy was seen to possess particular skills gleaned through her extensive experience. These skills were a benefit to her agency, as she was able to navigate the journey by containing and placating the agency's potentially vocal and problematic clients.

It is standard for experienced surrogates—those who have successfully completed a surrogacy journey (marked by the birth of a live child)—to be offered and to receive higher fees than inexperienced ones due to both the fact that they have proved themselves (that is, they can get pregnant via IVF and release the child to the IPs) and the skills they have gleaned from their earlier journeys. So while women are not encouraged to think of themselves as workers, those with more work experience are valued and usually paid more. This highlights the fact that contradictions exist in how surrogates are socialized to think about money and their work and the demands placed on them by the industry. On one hand, women are strongly encouraged to deny the monetary benefits they accrue through surrogacy. The emphasis on altruism permeates all aspects of surrogacy—including recruitment materials (which advertise "giving the gift of life"), interactions with others (people who call them "saints" and "angels"), the language used within agencies (they receive "compensation," not a "paycheck"), and the feeling rules about money they are encouraged to follow.

On the other hand, surrogates enter into formalized legal contracts, and they are encouraged to seek legal counsel and to negotiate or agree to compensation packages and structured fee schedules. Though surrogates are not supposed to admit having a deep interest in money, surrogates strongly encourage each other to closely examine their contracts and compensation amounts. On online support group websites you can read posts from surrogates to each other urging women to understand their legal agreements and to demand appropriate packages to "protect their families" should "problems arise." One agency director, Cheryl Woodley, let me know that most of the women in her agency were very "clued in" when it came to their compensation. Unlike surrogates in previous generations, these "modern-day ladies" (as Cheryl referred to them) negotiate quickly, without hesitation. Cheryl, who has worked in surrogacy for decades, attributes this to a "new generation" of surrogate mothers—"the me generation," she called them. These women, she said, are "wonderful, generous women," but they are also most concerned with their own experiences of surrogacy, rather than those of their IPs. Cheryl characterized her contemporary surrogates as having the following mind-set: "This is *my* journey, *my* pregnancy, *my* story." She went on:

> The latest generation is very "me" oriented. In fact if you look at many of their blogs, a lot of the stories they talk about is their feelings, their desires. Very rarely do they say, "I feel so bad for my . . ." They'll say, "I had a miscarriage.

I'm devastated. It's terrible." They very rarely will say, "Oh my goodness, my poor couple is devastated. I wish they would get more counseling. This is the end of the road to them. What do they do now?" They touch on it, but they don't dwell on it because it's more about "me" than it ever is about "them."

This "me" orientation lends itself, Cheryl argued, to a deep knowledge about standard surrogate fees and compensation packages. Surrogates today "do a lot of research," they "pore over" their contracts, and "make sure it really, really works for them," Cheryl said. They are "generous" women, "not bad surrogates," because of this, Cheryl emphasized. But they are knowledgeable and interested in being protected and facilitating a certain type of experience for themselves. Because of this, Cheryl's agency sets standard fees for compensation. Negotiation still occurs, but Cheryl and her colleagues attempt to negotiate surrogates' fees before matching women with IPs. Other agencies are more loosely structured, allowing surrogates and IPs to negotiate fees themselves (most often through their lawyers or in counseling sessions).

Another important related money rule that can be found throughout the surrogacy world is that surrogates and IPs are not encouraged to discuss money directly (hence the lawyers and counselors), but rather to use the agency as a middleman to iron out any issues with compensation or reimbursement fees. This rule of surrogates and IPs avoiding money talk, Cheryl told me, was to protect the integrity of the surrogacy process. If IPs were privy to the extended negotiating of surrogates, according to Cheryl, they "will say, 'Why does she need this extra money?' and 'It's all about money!'" To avoid such problems between surrogates and IPs and ensure a framing of surrogacy as an altruistically driven exchange, as sacrifice, and as explicitly not work, Cheryl's agency and many others socialize both surrogates and IPs into thinking about their relationship as one occurring outside of the marketplace. This is enabled by the money rule that bans or dissuades IPs and surrogates from talking about money with each other.

Many of the surrogates I spoke with indicated that they were directly told not to talk money with their IPs. Martha Griffin, the counselor at a large agency, stated emphatically, "We don't let people talk about money directly." Most of the surrogates appreciated this. When I asked Rhonda Chapman, for example, if she ever talked with her IPs "about the costs of IVF and surrogacy," she replied: "No. And that's not something that you're supposed to do. When you go through the agency they've got certain rules and parameters, and you're not supposed to have those kind of discussions with the couple. I think because it keeps the relationship more personal, more about the pregnancy and the babies, as opposed to some kind of a business transaction." Rhonda's assessment that not discussing money was a strategy to keep "the relationship more personal . . . as opposed to some kind of business transaction" was the same interpretation of this rule given by other surrogates and professionals. I was told repeatedly that discussing money was uncomfortable for surrogates and would create divisions among IPs and surrogates, which would inhibit people from appreciating and enjoying the "true meaning of surrogacy." Amber Castillo, for example, told me: "I like that with the agency you never have to ask the couple anything about monetary [matters]. There's no awkwardness there." This, in fact, was one of the important reasons women tended to choose agency-brokered surrogacies instead of independent arrangements. In independent arrangements, surrogates and IPs must discuss money not only during the contract phase but throughout the journey, as fees are paid and issues arise. While several women reported that although they did not enjoy talking about money with their IPs, they were not uncomfortable doing so, the overwhelming majority of the surrogates in my study, who each had at least one agency-brokered journey, told me that they did not want to have to talk about money face to face with their IPs.

Recall that many of my participants expressed considerable guilt over the compensation they received, which they envisioned would only be exacerbated if they had to discuss money directly with their IPs. Though surrogates value the work they do and many participants argued that they deserve (and most do receive) monetary compensation for their efforts, they do not want to think about their IPs dispensing money directly to them. Part of this guilt was associated with the immense pleasure they derive from being surrogates; surrogacy was too enjoyable, in other words, to receive monetary compensation for it. As many surrogates establish deep connections with their IPs, they are also intimately aware of the financial burden of third-party pregnancy. Josephine Maselli, for example, told me: "I feel very guilty. I personally feel very guilty that [my IPs] compensated me for something that was such an amazing thing to be a part of anyway." Surrogates feel guilty about their role in their IPs' financial burden. Rosalyn Whelan told me that "not a lot of people really talk about" the guilt associated with compensation, but that it does not "necessarily go away the more experienced you are." She explained:

> I just think everyone at some point kind of goes through something or there's an incident of—they received a gift or they received money or something, and they just get this guilt. Even though you've agreed on it, it's like, why do you feel this way? There's always posts [online] like, "I feel so bad. I feel so guilty." Because it's just hard. It's hard to take from someone that you got so close with. Because you don't want to think of it like a business deal. But half of it is, and half of it isn't. And it's hard to remind yourself that yes, it is. [sighs] Argh. I don't even like to think about it!

Like Rosalyn, many of the women I spoke with told me that they "don't even like to think about" the "business" aspect of surrogacy or the fact that their fees are coming directly from their IPs. Most did not talk directly to their IPs about money. Most of those that did informed me that these were awkward situations and ones they tried to avoid. Most women appreciated the rule, then, about not discussing money with their IPs.

I did have several women in my study who first completed agency-brokered journeys and then went on to complete independent ones and, therefore, discussed money directly with their IPs. One of those women, Sandra Foster, explained: "I'm more comfortable working directly with somebody and some-body who is comfortable working directly with me. Why have somebody in the middle? Why? I know there's agencies that tell people, 'You're not allowed to talk about money.' You can't talk about money with your IPs, you have to talk about it with [the agency]. Then there's people who have been ripped off by agencies, and I know some of them [the agencies] are reputable, but some of them are not. I've worked for a couple agencies, so I know!" Like other women who worked independently, Sandra felt that surrogacy agencies were "rip-offs." She reported that agencies "don't do enough to validate getting paid the money they get paid. And it just seems like a rip-off." She went on: "But I suppose if IPs felt more com-fortable with having that middleman, then that would be good for them. And some surrogates feel better with that, too. I'm just not one of them. I just would rather do it myself. We get to know each other better. It just works out that way." While Sandra and several other women became comfortable talking directly with their IPs about compensation, most surrogates reported an appreciation for the money rule that discouraged such conversations.

This particular money rule of surrogates and IPs not discussing money directly with each other is facilitated by—or perhaps dictates—the structure of fee payment in many agencies. Most agencies not only do not allow surrogates and IPs to discuss money, they do not allow money to pass directly from IPs to surrogates. Agencies serve as the middleman for both negotiations about and payments of money. Agencies do this by creating escrow accounts into which IPs deposit their fees and from which surrogates are paid. Some surrogates receive monthly compensation, while others receive their checks by the trimes-ter. Many agencies structure payment to coincide with important events in the surrogacy journey: the transfer, confirmation of pregnancy, confirmation of fetal heartbeat, movement from one trimester to the next, and birth. Particular procedures also have attached payments: if a surrogate undergoes amniocen-tesis she often receives a bonus check; if the IPs choose to selectively reduce, she receives another check. The payments are scheduled in specific ways, often spread throughout the journey, to avoid the appearance of payment for the child. Allowing the agencies to handle the money and negotiate any discrepancies allows surrogate-IP relationships and interactions to remain seemingly outside the world of commerce.

As I discussed above, some surrogates feel so guilty they refuse compensation or ask for reduced fees. While the majority of women in my study expressed a sense of guilt about compensation, all but one of them received fees—and most received the standard market amounts for their communities (there are variations by state and by agency)—for their work as surrogates. This was, in fact, another common money rule: surrogates should receive compensation for their services. Though some women refuse compensation, both surrogates and professionals with whom I spoke emphasized the importance of payment for surrogacy.

Surrogates reported compensation was an important insurance policy to assist their families should problems arise in their journeys. This can be seen in Treena Winmer's comments when she was explaining how much she made on her first surrogacy journey: "But my first journey was for a first-time surrogate, was like starting out at—I don't know. You start out at $18,000. And it was just something I wanted so bad, and I said, 'No, I'll do it for $10,000!' And if I could go back, I would do it for free because [those IPs] are just fabulous! I just love them to death. Wonderful! But I still need to make sure that my family was taken care of should I have to go on bed rest."

Notice how quickly Treena tempers her enthusiastic statement of "I would do it for free!" with "but I still need to make sure that my family was taken care of." As discussed in the previous chapter, most surrogates justify their compensation by thinking about it in the context of their families and by using the money on their families (especially their children). Surrogacy agencies, in fact, encourage women to think about compensation as a special thank-you gift to their children and husbands for taking mom away from them for so long. Martha Griffin emphasizes to her surrogates how important marking their journeys were by spending some of their compensation "doing something [they] wouldn't normally do"—such as taking their family to SeaWorld or Disney World or simply "tak[ing] everyone to Ben and Jerry's that night"—rather than only paying off credit cards. Doing something special, Martha told me, helps surrogates gain "closure" and "feelings of appreciation."

While counselors and agency directors emphasized the importance of closure for the emotional state of surrogates, paying compensation also gives IPs closure from the relationship, if they so desire. This is because compensation allows surrogacy to be conceptualized and experienced as a gift exchange rather than as a one-sided sacrifice. Building on the work of Claude Lévi-Strauss (1969) and Marcel Mauss (1954), Richard Titmuss emphasized in his seminal work on blood donation that gift relationships should be—and are—reciprocal: "To give is to receive—to compel some return or create some obligation—either in the form of a similar or different material gift or in the overt expression of sentiment, pleasure or pain, manifested in physical acts of behavior on the part of the recipient. No such gift is or can be utterly detached, disinterested or impersonal. Each carries message and motives in its own language" (1977, 277). While the donation of the uterus and the birthing services for the child are conceptualized in surrogacy culture as a gift, so too is compensation. Without compensation, IPs would be entirely obligated and beholden to surrogates, who could then demand "overt expression[s] of sentiment." This, in any case, is the fear of agency directors, many of whom insist that their surrogates accept compensation to protect their IPs from the possibility of never-ending obligation. Compensation is essential, therefore, to help smooth the transition out of the surrogate-IP relationship, if so desired. According to the surrogacy professionals with whom I spoke, compensation provides surrogates with a sign of proper sentiment and appreciation from their IPs. It serves as a gift to their families to help assuage any residual guilt for the time investment of surrogacy participation. And it allows IPs to sever or reduce ties with their surrogates without feelings of guilt, if they so desire. It is also essential in the recruitment of new surrogates. Without compensation for surrogates, the surrogacy industry in the United States might grind to a halt.

Thinking about money, talking about compensation, considering the work involved, and acknowledging the skills garnered through surrogacy are loaded issues in the surrogacy community. Surrogates are trained and socialized to both accept compensation and subscribe to nonmarket framings of that money. This is the heart of the contemporary dilemma of surrogacy: compensation is essential to the industry, and yet it is what makes the industry most vulnerable to criticism and attack.

MONEY RULES IN CONTEXT

The money rules of surrogacy in the United States are shaped by particular ideas about reproductive work that differ from attitudes about such work and compensation found in other national contexts. For example, as shown earlier in this book, poor women motivated by remuneration are explicitly recruited in India (DasGupta and Das Dasgupta 2014a; Hochschild 2012; Rudrappa 2012). Their desire for money is viewed as what enables them to engage in and to be recruited for surrogacy, which is a highly stigmatized activity, often equated to sex work, in that country (Nayak 2014). Compensation is not seen in India as inhibiting the proper functioning of surrogacy arrangements or leading to surrogates' disappointment. On the contrary, poverty and the desire for money enable and justify surrogacy in India. Likewise, Elly Teman (2010, 208) argues that in the Israeli context there is little stigma attached to compensation for women who birth children for others. She described 70 percent of her sample of twenty-six Israeli surrogates as lower class or very poor, living on "welfare stipends or government aid of some sort" (ibid., 24). Israeli surrogates were "up-front" in their acknowledgment to Teman that their motivations were "primarily economic" (ibid., 208). Teman explained that the women in her study "also expressed the desire to help a childless couple, but altruism was not considered a strong enough reason to motivate them to become surrogates" (ibid.). Only in the United States are surrogates required to demonstrate financial stability. They are also under tremendous pressure to deny the desire for and benefits of compensation in ways that surrogates in other countries are not.

Unlike in India and Israel, in the United States engaging in reproduction for money is often framed as greedy and indicative of negative character traits. This framing is exemplified in the phrase "renting a womb," which is a popular one in surrogacy discourse. It is used in stories in the media, in academic articles, and on television talk shows by everyone from academics to Oprah. It is so common because it captures perfectly the major cultural dilemma of contemporary surrogacy—namely, whether gestating and birthing babies should be commercialized. There is a deep cultural unease with the exchange of money for pregnancy, let alone cash for babies (which is illegal in every state). "Renting a womb" captures this unease and is often used to negatively characterize women seeking monetary compensation for bearing children. "Renting a womb" is also used to highlight the dystopian character of contemporary society. The image of a bare pregnant belly (or bellies) sometimes accompanies stories that include the phrase. Many times the final touch is a barcode imprinted across the taut skin. The image is meant to provoke or incense viewers, pushing them to wonder "how could women do that?" and "how could we as society allow this to happen?"

As explored in this book, surrogacy has flourished in the United States because of medical advances (for example, artificial insemination and IVF) coupled with a neoliberal market, pronatalism, and an unease with government interference in private matters of the family. Though the surrogacy market has been under construction and in expansion for the past three decades, societal acceptance and understanding of its arrangements have not kept pace (Markens 2007). While there is cultural variation in people's response to surrogacy, with some celebrating and applauding these arrangements (especially those who work in the field or who have benefited from surrogacy), a deep cultural unease remains. This unease centers on commodification. As I have argued in this book, an obscuring of surrogacy work is enacted by the surrogacy industry, surrogacy professionals, IPs, surrogates' families, and surrogates themselves due to that ongoing unease with commercialized third-party reproduction. The obscuring of surrogacy labor is necessary because of the dominant ideologies in US society that surrogacy confronts.

The first ideology that surrogacy challenges is a decidedly pronatalist position that posits women should birth children and should mother the children they birth. This ideology is based on notions of traditional motherhood: that women possess an intrinsic need to mother, they have inherent bonds with the children they gestate and birth, and they possess innate skills as mothers (Glenn 1994; M. Nelson 1990; Russo 1976). Though these notions are applied to all women, historically that need to mother has been explicitly exploited or curbed in poor women of color and encouraged among the white middle class (Cahn 2009; Gordon 1974; Jones 1985; Solinger 2005).

On a symbolic level, womanhood is tightly correlated with motherhood—or, as Evelyn Nakano Glenn puts it, "mothering and gender are closely intertwined: each is a constitutive element of the other" (1994, 3). The effect of this ideology can be seen in the challenges faced by women who choose to remain childless (Campbell 2003; Gillespie 2003; K. Park 2002). As Gayle Letherby notes, "motherhood is still a primary role for women and women who do not mother either biologically or socially are often stereotyped as either desperate or selfish" (2002, 7). This ideology can also be applied to women who are characterized as mothering poorly. Proper motherhood and natural womanhood are so tightly bound together that women who neglect or abuse their children are characterized as not only as unwomanly but also as unnatural, animal-like, and even monstrous (D. Roberts 1997 and 2002). In a strongly pronatalist culture such as that of the United States, good women are good mothers (Lovett 2007; Russo 1976).

This intrinsic motherhood in women, conceptualized as natural and sacred, is understood to exist outside the realm of the public and inside the private environment of the family. As Glenn explains, "mothering in Western culture has been defined in terms of binary oppositions between male-female, mind-body, nature-culture, reason-emotion, public-private, and labor-love. Mothering has been assigned to the subordinate poles of these oppositions: thus it is viewed as flowing from 'natural' female attributes, located only in the private sphere of family and involving strong emotional attachment and altruistic motives" (1994, 13). This ideology relies on false dichotomies not only between men and women but also between private and public, placing reproductive labor firmly within the family, the private, and the uncommercial. It is not that this ideology dictates a disavowal of women's labor within families. On the contrary, women's labor in the home is often valorized, identified as specialized female work. This ideology positions that reproductive labor is unpaid work engaged in because of love, familial commitment, and women's altruistic leanings.

As explored above in this book, the close correlation of proper womanhood with good mothering shapes norms regarding women and work, encouraging guilt among women over their paid labor. While the majority of women in the United States today, even those with young children, work outside of the home, strong gender norms and socialization efforts remain regarding women's nurturing role of altruism, selflessness, and caring for others, all of which emphasize the importance of women's family activities over those associated with their work lives (Damaske 2011). As examined in this book, surrogates reported feelings of guilt over their working lives as surrogates in large part because of the ways surrogacy pulled them from their families and because of their own enjoyment of surrogacy activities.

Dominant ideologies of motherhood place pregnancy and birth as exist-ing outside the market, as activities culturally framed as private, familial, and natural. Surrogacy challenges these understandings of motherhood as it takes pregnancy and birth outside the private, familial realm and commodifies those skills in a market arena. Surrogacy defies the natural bonds that are thought to occur via the process of gestation and birth, therefore according surrogates a position like that of women who choose not to mother and those who are seen as not mothering well: unnatural women (E. Roberts 1998; Teman 2010). Thus, the marketing of reproduction is seen as not only intruding into the private family realm but also often as immoral.

It is important to emphasize the gendered nature of these dominant ideolo-gies regarding reproductive labor. The work on gamete donation is helpful here, as it offers a gender comparison of reproductive workers in ways that surrogacy cannot. As Rene Almeling (2007 and 2011) argues in her work on egg and sperm donation, the particular framing of compensated reproductive work as somehow wrong is differentiated by gender in the United States and is specific to women. Almeling shows that both male and females donating gametes report both finan-cial and altruistic motivations, but only women are encouraged to emphasize the giving nature of their actions and to downplay the monetary incentives. For male sperm donors, there is no such pressure. Like surrogacy, egg donation for women is framed within the reproductive market as an altruistic gift, not a part-time job, "while men are informed of [sperm donation] as a job opportu-nity" (Almeling 2007, 328). As Almeling's work on gamete donors demonstrates, there is an intense cultural unease with women, but not with men, engaging in reproductive work for pay. This unease with female reproductive work and with the workers themselves—with the commodification of what is understood to be natural, familial, and private—is shaped by strong gender norms about women and their symbolic relationship to children and families.

However, cultural unease with the merger of commerce and reproduction alone does not fully explain the elaborate machinations involved in obscuring surrogate labor. Pregnancy and birth are big business in the United States—not only or even primarily because of surrogacy, but also because of the medicaliza-tion of birth (Block 2008; Davis-Floyd 2004; Spar 2006). Surrogacy accounts for a trifle of the revenue generated from the "approximately four million annual births" in the United States, which was recently estimated to be "well over $50 billion" (Rosenthal 2013). While surrogacy can run upward of $150,000 per journey, "the average total price charged for pregnancy and newborn care" for a non-surrogacy pregnancy and birth in the United States is "about $30,000 for a vaginal delivery and $50,000 for a C-section," with patients "with insur-ance pay[ing] out of pocket an average of $3,400" (ibid.). Though surrogacy is a growing market and is prohibitively expensive for many, it is minute—in terms of both number of cases per year and total revenue—compared to other forms of assisted reproduction and to pregnancy and birth without the use of assisted reproductive technology (ART).

Pregnancy and birth are intimate familial activities, but they are also commercial industries in the United States. There is a spectrum of commercialization (with surrogacy at the most commercialized end), not a false dichotomy between private regular birth and surrogacy. The unease with—the moral dilemma related to—the commercialization of reproduction is particularly acute with surrogacy. Protests against the monetary costs of pregnancy and birth in the United States often center on rising medical costs and problems with the institution of medicine, not on the intersection of commerce and reproduction per se. Though there is a home-birth movement in the United States, arguments against the commercialization of reproduction are often reserved for assisted reproduction—especially third-party pregnancy, in which individual reproductive workers profit monetarily in addition to revenue being generated for the medical community.

There is cultural unease with the way in which assisted reproduction, especially surrogacy, appears to commodify not only pregnancy but also humans, via the bodies of unrelated individuals. As Linda Layne notes, surrogacy raises a "discomfort with the commodification of life" in the same way that commercial adoption does (1999, 3). In modern US society there is revulsion at the idea of exchanging money for people. Igor Kopytoff notes that this revulsion can be traced to the particular history of slavery in the United States. "Contemporary Americans," he contends, "are strikingly sensitive to the morality of any social arrangement that may be taken to be reminiscent of slavery" (2004, 272). This helps explain the structure of contemporary adoption and surrogacy, in which there are elaborate procedures and checks to ensure that the money given by IPs not be construed as payment for the children but for services provided (Yngvesson 2004). Additionally, framing the adoptee or surro-child as a gift (from the birth mother, surrogate or God), rather than as a thing given in an economic exchange, emphasizes the agency of birth mothers and surrogates, thus reducing the discomfort over the potential interpretation of money for humans and the exploitation of birthing women.

In addition to norms against the exchange of money for humans, there are norms against the intersection of the market and the body (Kopytoff 2004). This can be seen in the unease with commodifying matter that comes from the human body—such as blood (Titmuss 1997), organs and tissues (Waldby and Mitchell 2006), breast milk (Weaver and Williams 1997), and gametes (Almeling 2011). We can no longer legally buy people, organs, or blood in the United States; their sale was seen to be "ultimately degrading for society as a whole" (Le Grand 1997, 334). But there is a thriving black or gray market for some of them, especially in other countries (Briggs 2012). Surrogacy and adoption butt up against both the cultural edict against commodifying humans and the knowledge of the existence of this black or gray market. Just as some adoptive mothers are asked about their daughters "How much did she cost?" (Jacobson 2008, 146–47), surrogates told me they are asked "How much do you make?" These questions raise the issue of placing a price tag on human life, on a child, in these markets. The money rules applied to surrogates—not talking about money, not being motivated by money, not receiving money directly from the IPs—are techniques used to distance surrogacy from commodification and the gray market in babies.

Ideologies of women and work and of reproduction, as well as edicts against the commodification of babies and the body, all converge in the topic of surrogacy in the United States. The money rules of surrogacy exist to make surrogacy less problematic by attempting to separate it from the ideas of baby selling, exploitation of women, the market in babies, and unnatural women. The money rules also encourage women to properly orient themselves toward pregnancy, birth, and children. The rules are essential to the obscuring of surrogate labor. The proper orientation of surrogates toward surrogacy—thinking with the heart, instead of the head—and obscuring surrogacy labor as work are so important to the continuing functioning of surrogacy, its social acceptance, and the recruitment of new women as reproductive workers, that I would argue that the surrogacy industry in the United States rotates around these particular issues.

Conclusion

Commercial surrogacy is a small but thriving market in the United States and, I imagine, it will continue to remain so—even with the advent of successful uterine transplant births. A large part of the success of surrogacy in the United States is because most other advanced industrialized nations ban or severely limit commercial surrogacy and because there are only several industrializing nations that have organized surrogacy industries (for example, India, Mexico, and Thailand). Some critics of surrogacy argue for a ban on commercial surrogacy in the United States similar to those that have been adopted in other nations. The American Society for Reproductive Medicine and some of the surrogacy professionals I interviewed advocate more regulation instead. Federal regulation would give surrogacy a professional legitimacy, I was told by the agency directors with whom I spoke, and would help ferret out unscrupulous practitioners and problematic surrogates. Israel, for example, has a state-run surrogacy program that institutionalizes cultural rules, and this is partly why the practice is relatively accepted (Teman 2010).

However, federal regulation in the United States would require a discussion of surrogacy at the federal level, which, as Debora Spar (2006) notes, the federal government would be reluctant to engage in due to the neoliberal underpinnings supporting the surrogacy market in the United States and the religious and ethical debates that would ensue. Surrogacy regulation currently remains at the state level, and the tenor of state discussions has increasingly leaned toward supporting the surrogacy industry, not limiting its reach. The medical market for reproduction is enormous in the United States, as is the pressure—especially for white, middle-class women—to procreate. So while there is cultural unease with surrogacy, there are also strong pressures to allow it to exist and expand. This is one of the important contradictions shaping contemporary surrogacy. There is demand and support for surrogacy, yet it remains controversial, arousing deep-seated anxieties about the intersection of the market and reproduction, women and work, and the commodification of humans and their biological products.

The cultural anxiety about surrogacy belies the numbers of annual surrogacy births, which are minuscule compared to other forms of alternative family formation arrangements, advanced reproductive procedures, and unassisted births (Markens 2007; Spar 2006). While there are roughly four million births per year in the United States, and approximately 1.5 percent of them are via ART, the number of surrogacy births is estimated at only around 1,500 per year (Centers for Disease Control and Prevention 2015; Hamilton and Sutton 2013; Kleinpeter 2002; Markens 2007; Shanley 2001; Teman 2010).

It is obviously not the numbers of women gestating and bearing children for others that holds the public's imagination; sells newspapers, magazines, and books; and creates such controversy. It is not even the development of a surrogacy industry per se. Rather, it is the fact that there are women who engage in surrogacy for money. There is a culturally untenable marriage of womb and money in surrogacy in the United States that has captured the public's fascination since the Baby M case in the late 1980s. This unease has played a large role in shaping popular understandings of surrogacy; the structure of the surrogacy market; and the experiences of surrogates and their families, IPs, and surrogacy professionals. This unease has given birth to a culture of surrogacy—norms of behavior, values, rhetoric, marketing techniques, and terminology. Surrogacy culture operates to protect the practice of surrogacy, largely through industry and community regulation of surrogates' behavior and through particular framings of their work. At the same time, surrogacy is celebrated, especially by those who have been positively touched by this practice. In my interviews with surrogates, IPs, family members, and professionals, it became clear to me how deeply connected people become to surrogacy and how much positive meaning it can hold in their lives—not only because of the birth of children, but also because of the deep satisfaction women derive from participating in surrogacy. Surrogates reported that they love their work and attain much joy and satisfaction from it. Surrogacy is work, and much of that work—including protecting the industry from scrutiny—falls on the backs of the surrogates. As I have explored in this book, that work is more than simply hidden: it is deliberately obscured to make it culturally palatable.

The obscuring of surrogate labor allows surrogacy to function in the United States, yet I would argue that it poses potential costs for individual surrogates, IPs, and women more generally. Surrogacy represents the extreme of female-oriented occupations, matched only perhaps by wet nurses in centuries past. Men simply cannot be surrogates. As I have explored in this book, similar to other service professions dominated by women (for example, child care, elder care, and nursing) there is the potential for depressed wages and labor exploitation in surrogacy. None of the surrogates in my study indicated that they thought the market rates for surrogate compensation were too low (though some did wish that they had altered the fees they had agreed on). However, the pressure to think this way is high, as the money rules serve to temper any potential demands for higher compensation packages. Although no woman reported that she felt exploited due to her participation in surrogacy, the structure of the industry and the culture of surrogacy in the United States cannot be thought of as free from potential exploitation and the negative effects of inequality for surrogates, IPs, and women generally.

The surrogacy fee structure currently prices many people out of this form of infertility treatment. Like other reproductive technologies, surrogacy is largely available only to people with enough disposable income or good enough credit to afford the high prices. The high cost of surrogacy is not due solely to the compensation surrogates receive (in contrast to the way it is often presented in the media) but rather to the combined medical, legal, and agency fees that often must be paid for multiple attempts. It is also due to the fact that "only a few states require private insurance coverage for infertility care, and Medicaid does not cover [such] treatment" (Bell 2014, 7). Depending on the total cost of a surrogacy journey, which can be more than $150,000, the $20,000–$35,000 that surrogates make does not account for the majority of revenue generated from surrogacy. The media focus on and public fascination with surrogates' wages rather conveniently diverts attention from the high cost of infertility treatment and the profit of medical professionals and surrogacy agencies. A more open discussion of the work involved in surrogacy—and the work distribution across different players—might open up greater consideration of the costs of infertility medical treatment and the unequal access to it of the estimated 12 percent of the American population of reproductive age experiencing infertility (American Society for Reproductive Medicine 2010, 4; Spar 2006, 3).

Obscuring the work of surrogacy also does not allow for recognition of the intensity of the medical protocol involved in surrogacy. Several women expressed concerns about the potential long-term effects of the medicines they took on their journeys, but most did not. Those who did discuss their concerns with their REs or obstetrician-gynecologists were told that the long-term effects were currently unknown, which appeared to satisfy them—at least, enough that they continued with treatment. Greater acknowledgment of surrogacy as work might encourage greater critical thinking about the working conditions of surrogates, including surrogacy's potential immediate and long-term physical toll on them.

The obscuring of surrogacy work encourages a framing of surrogacy as low-skilled, innately rote labor. Recognition of the work of surrogacy would not only acknowledge the skill-based work in which surrogates are engaged but might also encourage discussion of the work of pregnancy and birth more generally. If surrogates are paid for their work to birth children, perhaps all women should receive some benefit—such as paid and substantial maternity leave—for doing so. Greater recognition of surrogacy labor might also encourage discussion of the infertility industry and ways that society can support all women gestating and birthing children, regardless of their genetic connection to or their intended social mothering of those children.

Notes

ACKNOWLEDGMENTS

1. I use the term "surrogate" rather than "carrier," a term that has gained some popularity among surrogacy professionals, because it is the term the women in my study used to refer to themselves.

CHAPTER 1 — CONCEPTIONS

1. All names of study participants, including intended parents, surrogates, and surrogacy professionals (attorneys, physicians, psychologists, and agency employees) are pseudonyms.

2. *Skinner v. Oklahoma*, 316 U.S. 535, 541 (1942).

3. At the age of eighteen, Melissa Stern (formerly known as Baby M) terminated Whitehead's maternal rights and formalized her adoption by Elizabeth Stern.

CHAPTER 2 — MAKING REPRODUCTION PROFITABLE

1. Traditional surrogacy still exists today but has largely been replaced by gestational arrangements.

2. According to the State of Michigan Department of Human Services, "prior to 1995, Michigan was one of one of very few states that required a court termination of the rights of a child's parents before the child could be placed in a home for the purpose of adoption. Michigan prohibited the parents of a child from consenting to the adoption of their child by an unrelated, prospective adoptive parent." In 1995, changes were made that allowed for "a 'temporary placement' of a child in a prospective adoptive home immediately following birth, while the legal proceedings are being completed" (n.d.).

3. In the early 1980s it was illegal in at least twenty-four states for birth mothers to receive compensation in an adoption (Andrews 1984).

4. It was this issue, for example, that brought surrogacy to the Michigan State Supreme Court in 1981 in *Doe v. Kelley*, in which the court found that surrogacy contracts violated Michigan adoption law and thus were illegal (Butzel 1987).

5. In New York and Washington, altruistic surrogacy—that which does not involve compensation—is allowed and not criminalized. In Michigan, all forms of surrogacy are unenforceable.

6. In August 2012, New Jersey Governor Chris Christie vetoed a surrogacy bill that would have recognized surrogate arrangements and provided legal standards and safeguards.

7. California was a pioneer in surrogacy legislation. In the early 1990s a case brought before the California Supreme Court, *Johnson v. Calvert*, helped establish legal precedent for surrogacy. The case involved a black gestational carrier, a white intended father, and a Filipina intended mother and "marked the first time in US history that surrogacy had been declared enforceable and not contrary to public policy" (Markens 2007, 46).

8. It is not uncommon for IPs who live in states that have no protection for surrogacy arrangements to contract with surrogates who lives in surrogacy-friendly states. It is the state in which the surrogate birth takes place that matters in terms of protection.

9. This may change, of course, given the recent ruling by the US Supreme Court in *Obergefell v. Hodges* that states cannot ban same-sex marriage.

10. Initially, ICSI was used only if there were problems with the sperm, but it is now a common procedure accompanying IVF (Centers for Disease Control and Prevention 2013a).

11. The hormone hCG is produced in pregnancy.

12. Many of the surrogates in my study spoke of being "obsessed" with determining whether or not the transfer was a success, which was displayed through their use of home-pregnancy tests. Surrogates refer to the use of home pregnancy tests as "POAS," which stands for "peeing on a stick." Some called themselves "POAS-aholics" or "POAS obsessed."

13. There is, of course, variation in this sequence across individuals.

14. California now requires this for IPs and surrogates covered under Section 769 of the state's Family Code.

15. Before TRICARE, the health care program for active and retired US military personnel and their families, added a surrogacy exclusion, military wives were viewed as particularly suitable for surrogacy work due to their extensive medical coverage (among other reasons).

CHAPTER 3 — LABORING TO CONCEIVE

1. Using the class categories conceptualized by Annette Lareau (2003), Margaret Nelson (2010), and Michael Zweig (2000), I relied most heavily on education and power or authority in occupation in determining class. I define "middle-class households" as those in which at least one parent (either the surrogate or her spouse or partner) is employed and works in an occupation that is managerial or has some level of authority and requires a bachelor's degree or advanced skill set. I define "working-class or lower-middle-class households" as those in which at least one parent is employed and works in an occupation that has little authority and does not require an advanced skill set (none of the adults in this category in my sample had a college degree). I define "professional middle-class households" as those in which at least one parent has educational credentialing beyond a bachelor's degree, works in an occupation that requires an advanced degree, and has a high level of autonomy and authority (examples would be attorneys, physicians, and professors).

2. My source for the number of articles was LexisNexis, which I searched using the terms "surrogate motherhood" and "surrogacy."

CHAPTER 4 — MANAGING RELATIONS

1. Interestingly, IMs who purchase donor eggs they then gestate themselves often argue that it is the process of gestation and giving birth that creates motherhood. In those situations, pregnancy is privileged as a sacred act of motherhood; while in surrogacy, it is the dominance of genetics or intent that serves that purpose, with gestation and birth downplayed.

2. California has always been at the forefront of assisted reproduction for same-sex couples. With the amendment of the California Family Code that took effect on January 1, 2013, gestational surrogacy arrangements that follow certain procedures are legally protected regardless of the marital status or sexual orientation of the IPs. This differs from states like Texas, in which IPs must be married to enjoy the benefits of prosurrogacy law. It will be interesting to see how state surrogacy policy in Texas changes due to the June 26, 2015, US Supreme Court ruling in *Obergefell v. Hodges* that the Constitution guarantees every US citizen, including gays and lesbians, the right to marry.

3. The concept of "womb envy" was originally developed by the psychologist Karen Horney to denote the envy men have for women's ability to gestate and give birth: "Horney explained that it is just as likely that men have womb envy as women would have penis envy because it is women who are able to bring life into the world. To Horney, men compensate for their inability to produce life through the womb by their excessive efforts to be productive in the world of work" (Aldridge et al. 2014, 34). The surrogacy community has adapted Horney's concept to refer to infertile women's envy of other women's reproductive capabilities.

4. In my interviews, I was told about cases in which IPs have refused their intended children. Several such cases were discussed with me by agency directors. In one memorable case I was told about, the surro-baby was allegedly refused because he had Down syndrome. According to my informant, the agency helped facilitate the child's adoption.

5. Though this is a stated requirement of some agencies, if IPs refuse to abide by this requirement there is nothing agencies can do—outside of refusing to work with them again or scolding them.

6. This helps explain the devastation surrogates feel when their IPs do not attend the birth.

CHAPTER 5 — WORKING FROM HOME

1. Of course, in independent arrangements IPs can choose to work with whomever they desire—including women who have not previously given birth.

References

ABC News. 2014. "'Social Surrogacy' an Option for Moms-to-Be Who Shun Pregnancy." April 18. Accessed June 12, 2015. http://abcnews.go.com/blogs/lifestyle/2014/04/social-surrogacy-an-option-for-moms-to-be-who-shun-pregnancy/.

Abdalla, H. I., M. E. Wren, A. Thomas, and L. Korea. 1997. "Age of the Uterus Does Not Affect Pregnancy or Implantation Rates: A Study of Egg Donation in Women of Different Ages Sharing Oocytes from the Same Donor." *Human Reproduction* 12 (4): 827–29.

Abel, Emily. 2000. "A Historical Perspective on Care." In *Care Work: Gender, Labor, and the Welfare State*, edited by Madonna Harrington Meyer, 8–14. New York: Routledge.

Ademec, Christine, and Laurie C. Miller. 2007. *The Encyclopedia of Adoption*. 3rd ed. New York: Facts of File.

Aldridge, Jerry, Jennifer L. Kilgo, and Grace Jepkemboi. 2014. "Four Hidden Matriarchs of Psychoanalysis: The Relationship of Lou von Salome, Karen Horney, Sabina Spielrein and Anna Freud to Sigmund Freud." *International Journal of Psychology and Counseling* 6 (4): 32–39.

Allen, Anita L. 1988. "Colloquy: In re Baby M. Privacy, Surrogacy, and the Baby M Case." *Georgetown Law Journal* 76 (1759): 1–27.

Almeling, Rene. 2007. "Selling Genes, Selling Gender: Egg Agencies, Sperm Banks, and the Medical Market in Genetic Material." *American Sociological Review* 72 (3): 319–40.

―――. 2011. *Sex Cells: The Medical Market for Eggs and Sperm*. Berkeley: University of California Press.

American Society for Reproductive Medicine. n.d. "Q06: Is In Vitro Fertilization Expensive?" Accessed June 12, 2015. http://www.asrm.org/detail.aspx?id=3023.

―――. 2010. "Oversight of Assisted Reproductive Technology." Accessed June 10, 2015. http://www.asrm.org/uploadedFiles/Content/About_Us/Media_and_Public_Affairs/OversiteOfART%20%282%29.pdf.

―――. 2012a. "Recommendations for Practices Utilizing Gestational Carriers: An ASRM Practice Committee Guideline." *Fertility and Sterility* 97 (6): 1301–8.

―――. 2012b. "Third-Party Reproduction: A Guide for Patients." Accessed June 10, 2015. http://www.asrm.org/uploadedFiles/ASRM_Content/Resources/Patient_Resources/Fact_Sheets_and_Info_Booklets/thirdparty.pdf.

_____. 2012c. "Third-Party Reproduction: A Guide for Patients." Accessed June 15, 2010. http://www.asrm.org/uploadedFiles/ASRM_Content/Resources/Patient_Resources/ Fact_Sheets_and_Info_Booklets/thirdparty.pdf.

Andrews, Lori. 1984. "The Stork Market: The Law of the New Reproductive Technologies." *American Bar Association Journal* 70 (8): 50–56.

_____. 1989. *Between Strangers: Surrogate Mothers, Expectant Fathers, and Brave New Babies.* New York: Harper and Row.

_____. 1990. "Surrogate Motherhood: The Challenge for Feminists." In *Surrogate Motherhood: Politics and Privacy,* edited by Larry Gostin, 167–82. Bloomington: Indiana University Press.

_____. 1992. "Surrogacy Wars." *California Lawyer* 12 (10): 42–50.

Anleu, Sharyn Roach. 1992. "Surrogacy: For Love But Not for Money?" *Gender & Society,* 6 (1): 30–48.

Annas, George J. 1990. "Fairy Tales Surrogate Mothers Tell." In *Surrogate Motherhood: Politics and Privacy,* edited by Larry Gostin, 43–55. Bloomington: Indiana University Press.

Arieff, Adrienne. 2012. *The Sacred Thread: A True Story of Becoming a Mother and Finding a Family—Half a World Away.* New York: Crown.

Associated Press. 2014. "Woman Gives Birth after Womb Transplant, in Medical First." *Guardian,* October 3. Accessed June 21, 2015. http://www.theguardian.com/science/ 2014/oct/04/woman-gives-birth-womb-transplant-medical-first.

"Baby Is Born to Woman Who Received Womb Transplant." 2014. *Wall Street Journal,* October 4.

Bahn, David, Dara L. Havemann, and John Y. Phelps. 2010. "Reproduction beyond Menopause: How Old Is Too Old for Assisted Reproductive Technology?" *Journal of Assisted Reproduction and Genetics* 27 (7): 365–70.

Bailey, Alison. 2014. "Reconceiving Surrogacy: Toward a Reproductive Justice Account of Indian Surrogacy." In *Globalization and Transnational Surrogacy in India: Outsourcing Life,* edited by Sayantani DasGupta and Shamita Das Dasgupta, 23–44. Lanham, MD: Lexington.

Bartels, Dianne, Reinhard Preister, Dorothy Vawter, and Arthur Caplan. 1990. *Beyond Baby M: Ethical Issues in New Reproductive Techniques.* New York: Humana.

Becker, Gay. 2000. *The Elusive Embryo: How Women and Men Approach New Reproductive Technologies.* Berkeley: University of California Press.

Bell, Ann V. 2009. "'It's Way Out of My League': Low-Income Women's Experiences of Medicalized Infertility." *Gender & Society* 23 (5): 688–709.

_____. 2014. *Misconception: Social Class and Infertility in America.* New Brunswick, NJ: Rutgers University Press.

Berend, Zsuzsa. 2012. "The Romance of Surrogacy." *Sociological Forum* 27 (4): 913–36.

Berkowitz, Dana, and Marsiglio, William. 2007. "Gay Men: Negotiating Procreative, Father, and Family Identities." *Journal of Marriage and Family* 69 (2): 366–81.

Bianchi, Suzanne, John Robinson, and Melissa Milkie. 2006. *Changing Rhythms of American Family Life.* New York: Russell Sage.

Bijlsma-Frankema, Katinka, and Ana Cristina Costa. 2005. "Understanding the Trust-Control Nexus." *International Sociology* 20 (3): 259–82.

Block, Jennifer. 2008. *Pushed: The Painful Truth about Childbirth and Modern Maternity Care.* Cambridge, MA: Da Capo.

Boris, Eileen, and Rhacel Salazar Parrenas. 2010. Introduction to *Intimate Labors: Cultures, Technologies, and the Politics of Care*, edited by Eileen Boris and Rhacel Salazar Parrenas, 1–12. Stanford, CA: Stanford University Press.

Brännström, Mats, et al. 2015. "Livebirth after Uterus Transplantation." *Lancet*. 385 (9968): 607–16.

Braverman, Andrea Mechanick, and Stephen L. Corson. 1992. "Characteristics of Participants in a Gestational Carrier Program." *Journal of Assisted Reproduction and Genetics* 9 (4): 353–57.

Briggs, Laura. 2012. *Somebody's Children: The Politics of Transracial and Transnational Adoption*. Durham, NC: Duke University Press.

Bureau of Labor Statistics. 2013. *Women in the Labor Force: A Data Book*. BLS Report 1040. Accessed June 13, 2015. http://www.bls.gov/cps/wlf-databook-2012.pdf.

———. 2014. "Employment Characteristics of Families—2014." Accessed June 21, 2015. http://www.bls.gov/news.release/pdf/famee.pdf.

Butzel, Henry M. 1987. "The Essential Facts of the Baby M Case." In *On the Problem of Surrogate Parenthood: Analyzing the Baby M Case*, edited by Herbert Richardson, 7–20. Lewiston, NY: Edwin Mellen.

Cahn, Naomi R. 2009. *Test Tube Families: Why the Fertility Market Needs Regulation*. New York: New York University Press.

———. 2013. *The New Kinship: Constructing Donor Conceived Families*. New York: New York University Press.

Campbell, Annily. 2003. "Cutting Out Motherhood: Childfree Sterilized Women." In *Gender, Identity, and Reproduction: Social Perspectives*, edited by Sarah Earle and Gayle Letherby, 191–204. New York: Palgrave.

Celizic, Mike. 2007. "A Cautionary Tale for Couples Using Surrogates: One Couple Vows to Continue Battle with Woman Who Decided to Keep Baby." *Today Show*, October 23. Accessed June 10, 2015. http://www.today.com/id/21435600/ns/today-today_news/t/cautionary-tale-couples-using-surrogates/#.UXarDkqyLcw.

Centers for Disease Control and Prevention. 2011. "2011 Assisted Reproductive Technology National Summary Report." Accessed June 11, 2015. http://www.cdc.gov/art/ART2011/NationalSummary_index.htm.

———. 2013a. "2011 Data—Clinic Tables and Data Dictionary." Accessed July 15, 2015. http://www.cdc.gov/art/reports/archive.html.

———. 2013b. "Policy Documents: The Fertility Clinic Success Rate and Certification Act." Accessed June 11, 2015. http://www.cdc.gov/art/nas/policy.html.

———. 2015. "Assisted Reproductive Technology (ART)." Accessed July 13, 2015. http://www.cdc.gov/art/reports/index.html.

Charo, R. Alta. 1990. "Legislative Approaches to Surrogate Motherhood." In *Surrogate Motherhood: Politics and Privacy*, edited by Larry Gostin, 88–119. Bloomington: Indiana University Press.

Ciccarelli, Janice, and Linda Beckman. 2005. "Navigating Rough Waters: An Overview of Psychological Aspects of Surrogacy." *Journal of Social Issues* 61 (1): 21–43.

Cohen, Elizabeth. 2013. "Surrogate Offered $10,000 to Abort Baby." CNN, March 6. Accessed June 10, 2015. http://www.cnn.com/2013/03/04/health/surrogacy-kelley-legal-battle.

Colen, Shellee. 1995. "'Like a Mother to Them': Stratified Reproduction and West Indian Childcare Workers and Employers in New York." In *Conceiving the New World Order:*

The Global Politics of Reproduction, edited by Faye Ginsburg and Rayna Rapp, 78–102. Berkeley: University of California Press.

Coltrane, Scott, and Justin Galt. 2000. "The History of Men's Caring: Evaluating Precedents for Fathers' Family Involvement." In *Care Work: Gender, Labor, and the Welfare State*, edited by Madonna Harrington Meyer, 15–36. New York: Routledge.

Congregation for the Doctrine of the Faith. 1987. "Instructions on Respect for Human Life in Its Origin and on the Dignity of Procreation: Replies to Certain Questions of the Day." Accessed July 16, 2015. http://www.vatican.va/roman_curia/congregations/cfaith/documents/rc_con_cfaith_doc_19870222_respect-for-human-life_en.html.

Coontz, Stephanie. 1992. *The Way We Never Were: American Families and the Nostalgia Trap*. New York: Basic.

Corea, Gina. 1985. *The Mother Machine*. New York: Harper and Row.

Creative Family Connections. n.d. "Surrogacy Law by State." Accessed July 13, 2015. http://creativefamilyconnections.com/surrogacy-law-by-state/.

Damaske, Sarah. 2011. *For the Family: How Class and Gender Shape Women's Work*. New York: Oxford University Press.

Daniels, Arlene Kaplan. 1987. "Invisible Work." *Social Problems* 34 (5): 403–15.

DasGupta, Sayantani, and Shamita Das Dasgupta. 2014a. "Business as Usual? The Violence of Reproductive Trafficking in the Indian Context." In *Globalization and Transnational Surrogacy in India: Outsourcing Life*, edited by Sayantani DasGupta and Shamita Das Dasgupta, 179–96. Lanham, MD: Lexington.

_____, eds. 2014b. *Globalization and Transnational Surrogacy in India: Outsourcing Life*. Lanham, MD: Lexington.

_____. 2014c. Introduction to *Globalization and Transnational Surrogacy in India: Outsourcing Life*, edited by Sayantani DasGupta and Shamita Das Dasgupta, vii–xvii. Lanham, MD: Lexington.

Davis-Floyd, Robbie. 2004. *Birth as an American Rite of Passage*. Berkeley: University of California Press.

Delhi IVF. n.d. "Why India for Surrogate?" Accessed June 13, 2015. http://www.delhi-ivf.com/india_surrogacy.html.

DeVault, Marjorie. 1991. *Feeding the Family: The Social Organization of Caring as Gendered Work*. Chicago: University of Chicago Press.

Di Leonardo, Micaela. 1987. "The Female World of Cards and Holidays: Women, Families, and the Work of Kinship." *Signs* 12 (3): 440–53.

Dodson, Lisa, and Rebekah M. Zincavage. 2007. "'It's Like a Family': Caring Labor, Race, and Exploitation in Nursing Homes." *Gender & Society* 21 (6): 905–28.

Duffy, Mignon. 2005. "Reproducing Labor Inequalities: Challenges for Feminists Conceptualizing Care at the Intersections of Gender, Race, and Class." *Gender & Society* 19 (1): 66–82.

_____. 2011. *Making Care Count: A Century of Gender, Race, and Paid Care Work*. New Brunswick, NJ: Rutgers University Press.

Dunn, Patricia, Ione Ryan, and Kevin O'Brien. 1988. "College Students' Acceptance of Adoption and Five Alternative Fertilization Techniques." *Journal of Sex Research* 24 (1): 282–87.

Edelmann, Robert J. 2004. "Surrogacy: The Psychological Issues." *Journal of Reproductive and Infant Psychology* 22 (2): 123–36.

England, Paula. 2005. "Emerging Theories in Care Work." *Annual Review of Sociology* 31 (1): 381–99.

_____ and Nancy Folbre. 1999. "The Cost of Caring." *Annals of the American Academy of Political and Social Science* 561 (1): 39–51.

Ettorre, Elizabeth. 2002. *Reproductive Genetics, Gender, and the Body.* London: Routledge.

Evans, Mark I., Marion I. Kaufman, Anita J. Urban, David W. Britt, and John C. Fletcher. 2004. "Fetal Reduction from Twins to a Singleton: A Reasonable Consideration?" *Obstetrics & Gynecology* 104 (1): 102–9.

Federal Bureau of Investigation. 2011. "Surrogacy Scam: Preyed on Emotions of Vulnerable Victims." September 13. Accessed July 10, 2015. https://www.fbi.gov/news/stories/2011/september/surrogacy_091311.

_____. 2012. "Prominent Surrogacy Attorney Sentenced to Prison for Her Role in Baby-Selling Case." February 24. Accessed June 12, 2015. http://www.fbi.gov/sandiego/press-releases/2012/prominent-surrogacy-attorney-sentenced-to-prison-for-her-role-in-baby-selling-case.

_____. 2013a. "Modesto Surrogate Parenting Agency Owner Pleads Guilty in $2 Million Fraud Scheme." February 19. Accessed June 12, 2015. http://www.fbi.gov/sacramento/press-releases/2013/modesto-surrogate-parenting-agency-owner-pleads-guilty-in-2-million-fraud-scheme.

_____. 2013b. "Modesto Surrogate Parenting Agency Owner Sentenced to More Than Five Years in Prison in $2.4 Million Fraud Scheme." May 13. Accessed June 12, 2015. http://www.fbi.gov/sacramento/press-releases/2013/modesto-surrogate-parenting-agency-owner-sentenced-to-more-than-five-years-in-prison-in-2.4-million-fraud-scheme.

Field, Martha A. 1990. *Surrogate Motherhood: The Legal and Human Issues.* Cambridge, MA: Harvard University Press.

Fisher, Berenice. 1990. "Alice in the Human Services: A Feminist Analysis of Women in the Caring Professions." In *Circles of Care: Work and Identity in Women's Lives,* edited by Emily K. Abel and Margaret K. Nelson, 108–31. Albany: State University of New York Press.

Folbre, Nancy. 2001. *The Invisible Heart: Economics and Family Values.* New York: New Press.

Food and Drug Administration. 2007. "Guidance for Industry: Eligibility Determination for Donors of Human Cells, Tissues, and Cellular and Tissue-Based Products (HTC/Ps)." Accessed June 20, 2015. http://www.fda.gov/downloads/BiologicsBloodVaccines/GuidanceComplianceRegulatoryInformation/Guidances/CellularandGeneTherapy/ucm078703.pdf.

Franklin, Sarah. 1993. "Making Representations: The Parliamentary Debate on the Human Fertilisation and Embryology Act." In *Technologies of Procreation: Kinship in the Age of Assisted Conception,* edited by Jeanette Edwards, Sarah Franklin, Eric Hirsch, Frances Price, and Marilyn Strathern, 129–65. Manchester, UK: Manchester University Press.

_____. 1995. "Postmodern Procreation: A Cultural Account of Assisted Reproduction." In *Conceiving the New World Order: The Global Politics of Reproduction,* edited by Faye Ginsburg and Rayna Rapp, 323–45. Berkeley: University of California Press.

Fukuyama, Francis. 1995. *Trust: The Social Virtues and the Creation of Prosperity.* New York: Free Press.

_____. 1999. *The Great Disruption: Human Nature and the Reconstitution of Social Order.* New York: Free Press.

Gamson, William, and Gadi Wolfsfeld. 1993. "Movements and Media as Interacting Systems." *Annals of the American Academy* 528 (1): 114–25.

Gerstel, Naomi, and Natalia Sarkisian. 2006. "Marriage: The Good, the Bad, and the Greedy." *Contexts* 5 (4): 16–21.

Gillespie, Rosemary. 2003. "Childfree and Feminine: Understanding the Gender Identity of Voluntarily Childless Women." *Gender & Society* 17 (1): 122–36.

Glenn, Evelyn Nakano. 1992. "From Servitude to Service Work: Historical Continuities in the Racial Division of Paid Reproductive Labor." *Signs* 18 (1): 1–43.

———. 1994. "Social Constructions of Mothering: A Thematic Overview." In *Mothering: Ideology, Experience, and Agency*, edited by Evelyn Nakano Glenn, Grace Chang, and Linda Rennie Forcey, 1–29. New York: Routledge.

Goffman, Erving. 1959. *The Presentation of Self in Everyday Life*. New York: Anchor.

Gordon, Linda. 1974. "The Politics of Population: Birth Control and the Eugenics Movement." *Radical America* 8 (4): 61–98.

Goslinga-Roy, Gillian. 1998. "Naturalized Selves and Cyborg Bodies: The Case of Gestational Surrogacy." In *Biotechnology, Culture, and the Body*, edited by Paul Brodwin, 121–46. Bloomington: Indiana University Press.

———. 2000. "Body Boundaries, Fiction of the Female Self: An Ethnographic Perspective on Power, Feminism, and the Reproductive Technologies." *Feminist Studies* 26 (1): 113–40.

Gostin, Larry, ed. 1990. *Surrogate Motherhood: Politics and Privacy*. Bloomington: Indiana University Press.

Hamilton, Brady E., and Paul D. Sutton. 2013. "Recent Trends in Births and Fertility Rates through June 2013." National Center for Health Statistics, December 2013. Accessed June 23, 2015. http://www.cdc.gov/nchs/data/hestat/births_fertility_june_2013/births_ fertility_june_2013.pdf.

Hanafin, Hilary. 1984. "The Surrogate Mother: An Exploratory Study." PhD diss., California School of Professional Psychology.

Hansen, Karen. 2005. *Not-So-Nuclear Families: Class, Gender, and Networks of Care*. New Brunswick, NJ: Rutgers University Press.

Hartmann, Heidi. 1976. "Capitalism, Patriarchy, and Job Segregation by Sex." *Signs* 1 (3): 137–69.

———. 1981. "The Family as the Locus of Gender, Class, and Political Struggle." *Signs* 6 (3): 366–94.

Hartouni, Valerie. 1997. *Cultural Conceptions: On Reproductive Technologies and the Remaking of Life*. Minneapolis: University of Minnesota Press.

Hays, Sharon. 1996. *The Cultural Contradictions of Motherhood*. New Haven, CT: Yale University Press.

Healy, Kieran. 2006. *Altruism and the Market for Human Blood and Organs*. Chicago: University of Chicago Press.

Heck, Ramona, Alma Owen, and Barbara Rowe. 1995. *Home-Based Employment and Family Life*. Santa Barbara, CA: Praeger.

Hinson, Diane S., and Maureen McBrien. 2011. "Surrogacy across America: Both the Law and the Practice." *Family Advocate* 24 (2): 32–36.

Hochschild, Arlie Russell. 1979. "Emotion Work, Feeling Rules, and Social Structure." *American Journal of Sociology* 85 (3): 551–75.

———. 1983. *The Managed Heart: Commercialization of Human Feeling*. Berkeley: University of California Press.

_____. 1989. *The Second Shift*. New York: Avon.

_____. 1997. *The Time Bind: When Work Becomes Home and Home Becomes Work*. New York: Metropolitan.

_____. 2003. *The Commercialization of Intimate Life: Notes from Home and Work*. Berkeley: University of California Press.

_____. 2012. *The Outsourced Self: Intimate Life in Market Times*. New York: Metropolitan.

Holder, Angela R. 1990. "Surrogate Motherhood and the Best Interests of Children." In *Surrogate Motherhood: Politics and Privacy*, edited by Larry Gostin, 77–87. Bloomington: Indiana University Press.

Hondagneu-Sotelo, Pierrette. 2001. *Domestica: Immigrant Workers Cleaning and Caring in the Shadows of Influence*. Berkeley: University of California Press.

Jacobson, Heather. 2008. *Culture Keeping: White Mothers, International Adoption, and the Negotiation of Family Difference*. Nashville, TN: Vanderbilt University Press.

_____. 2014. "Framing Adoption: The Media and Parental Decision-Making." *Journal of Family Issues* 35 (5): 654–76.

Jones, Jacqueline. 1985. *Labor of Love, Labor of Sorrow: Black Women, Work, and the Family, From Slavery to the Present*. New York: Basic.

Katz, Patricia, Robert Nachtigall, and Jonathon Showstack. 2002. "The Economic Impact of the Assisted Reproductive Technologies." *Nature Cell Biology & Nature Medicine* 4 (Fertility Supplement): 29–32.

Ketchum, S. A. 1992. "Selling Babies and Selling Bodies." In *Feminist Perspectives in Medical Ethics*, edited by Helen Bequaert Holmes and Laura M. Purdy, 284–94. Bloomington: Indiana University Press.

Kleinpeter, Christine. 2002. "Surrogacy: The Parents' Story." *Psychological Reports* 91: 201–19.

Klymkowsky, Michael W., Kathy Garvin-Doxas, and Michael Zeilik. 2003. "Bioliteracy and Teaching Efficacy: What Biologists Can Learn from Physicists." *Cell Biology Education* 2:155–161.

Kopytoff, Igor. 2004. "Commoditizing Kinship in America." In *Consuming Motherhood*, edited by Janelle S. Taylor, Linda L. Layne, and Danielle F. Wozniak, 271–78. New Brunswick, NJ: Rutgers University Press.

Krishnan, Vijaya. 1994. "Attitudes toward Surrogate Motherhood in Canada." *Health Care for Women International* 15 (4): 333–57.

Lane, Melissa. 2003. "Ethical Issues in Surrogacy Arrangements." In *Surrogate Motherhood: International Perspectives*, edited by Rachel Cook and Shelley Day Sclater with Felicity Kaganas, 121–39. Oxford: Hart.

Lareau, Annette. 2003. *Unequal Childhoods: Class, Race, and Family Life*. Berkeley: University of California Press.

Larzelere, Robert, and Ted Huston. 1980. "The Dyadic Trust Scale: Toward Understanding Interpersonal Trust in Close Relationships." *Journal of Marriage and the Family* 42 (3): 595–604.

Layne, Linda. 1999. "The Child as Gift: New Directions in the Study of Euro-American Gift Exchange." In *Transformative Motherhood: On Giving and Getting in a Consumer Culture*, edited by Linda Layne, 1–27. New York: New York University Press.

Legislative Counsel of California. n.d. "California Family Code." Accessed June 27, 2015. http://www.leginfo.ca.gov/.html/fam_table_of_contents.html.

Le Grand, Julian. 1997. Afterword to Richard M. Titmuss, *The Gift Relationship: From Human Blood to Social Policy*, edited by Ann Oakley and John Ashton, 333–39. Expanded and updated edition. New York: New Press.

Letherby, Gayle. 2002. "Childless and Bereft? Stereotypes and Realities in Relation to 'Voluntary' and 'Involuntary' Childlessness and Womanhood." *Sociological Inquiry* 72 (1): 7–20.

Levine, Judith A. 2013. *Ain't No Trust: How Bosses, Boyfriends, and Bureaucrats Fail Low-Income Mothers and Why It Matters.* Berkeley: University of California Press.

Lévi-Strauss, Claude. 1969. *The Elementary Structures of Kinship.* Revised ed. Translated by James Harle Bell, John Richard von Sturmer, and Rodney Needham, editor. London: Eyre and Spottiswoode.

Lewin, Tamar. 2014. "Coming to U.S. for Baby, and Womb to Carry It." *New York Times,* July 6.

Lovett, Laura. 2007. *Conceiving the Future: Pronatalism, Reproduction, and the Family in the United States, 1890–1938.* Chapel Hill: University of North Carolina Press.

MacDonald, Cameron Lynn. 2010. *Shadow Mothers: Nannies, Au Pairs, and the Micropolitics of Mothering.* Berkeley: University of California Press.

Macklin, Ruth. 1990. "Is There Anything Wrong with Surrogate Motherhood? An Ethical Analysis." In *Surrogate Motherhood: Politics and Privacy,* edited by Larry Gostin, 136–50. Bloomington: Indiana University Press.

Madge, Varada. 2014. "Gestational Surrogacy in India: The Problem of Technology and Poverty." In *Globalization and Transnational Surrogacy in India: Outsourcing Life,* edited by Sayantani DasGupta and Shamita Das Dasgupta, 45–66. Lanham, MD: Lexington.

Malacrida, Claudia, and Tiffany Boulton. 2012. "Women's Perceptions of Childbirth 'Choices': Competing Discourses of Motherhood, Sexuality, and Selflessness." *Gender & Society* 26 (5): 748–72.

Malhotra, Deepak, and J. Keith Murnighan. 2002. "The Effects of Contracts on Interpersonal Trust." *Administrative Science Quarterly* 47 (3): 534–59.

Markens, Susan. 2007. *Surrogate Motherhood and the Politics of Reproduction.* Berkeley: University of California Press.

———. 2012. "The Global Reproductive Health Market: U.S. Media Framings and Public Discourse about Transnational Surrogacy." *Social Science & Medicine* 74 (11): 1745–53.

Martin, Joyce A., Brady E. Hamilton, Stephanie J. Ventura, Michelle J. K. Osterman, and T. J. Matthews. 2013. "Births: Final Data for 2011." *National Vital Statistics Reports* 62 (1). Accessed June 13, 2015. http://www.cdc.gov/nchs/data/nvsr/nvsr62/nvsr62_01.pdf#table01.

Maume, David, Rachel Sebastian, and Anthony Bardo. 2010. "Gender, Work-Family Responsibilities, and Sleep." *Gender & Society* 24 (6): 746–68.

Mauss, Marcel. 2000 [1954]. *The Gift.* Translated by W. D. Halls. London: Routledge.

McCormack, Karen. 2005. "Stratified Reproduction and Poor Women's Resistance." *Gender & Society* 19 (5): 660–79.

Meinke, Sue A. 1988. "Surrogate Motherhood: Ethical and Legal Issues." *Scope Note* 6. National Bioethics Research Library, Georgetown University. Accessed July 10, 2015. https://repository.library.georgetown.edu/bitstream/handle/10822/556906/sn6.pdf?sequence=1&isAllowed=y.

Michigan State University. 2007. "Scientific Literacy: How Do Americans Stack Up?" *ScienceDaily,* February 27. Accessed June 13, 2015. www.sciencedaily.com/releases/2007/02/070218134322.htm.

Morris, Theresa, and Katherine McInerney. 2010. "Media Representations of Pregnancy and Birth: An Analysis of Reality Television Programs in the United States." *Birth* 37 (2): 134–40.

Mundy, Liza. 2007. *Everything Conceivable: How Assisted Reproduction Is Changing Our World*. New York: Anchor.

Myers, Donald P. 1989. "After Baby M: Mary Beth Whitehead Has a New Storybook, and Some Tough Talk about Surrogate Motherhood." *Los Angeles Times*, March 6.

National Library of Medicine. 2011. "Leuprolide Injection." Accessed June 20, 2015. http://www.nlm.nih.gov/medlineplus/druginfo/meds/a685040.html.

National Science Foundation. 2004. "Science and Technology: Public Attitudes and Understanding." In *Science and Engineering Indicators 2004*, chapter 7. Accessed June 13, 2015. http://www.nsf.gov/statistics/seind04/c7/c7s2.htm.

Nayak, Preeti. 2014. "The Three Ms of Commercial Surrogacy in India: Mother, Money, and Medical Market." In *Globalization and Transnational Surrogacy in India: Outsourcing Life*, edited by Sayantani DasGupta and Shamita Das Dasgupta, 1–22. Lanham, MD: Lexington.

Nelson, Erin. 2013. "Global Trade and Assisted Reproductive Technologies: Regulatory Challenges in International Surrogacy." *Journal of Law, Medicine, & Ethics*, 41 (1): 240–53.

Nelson, Margaret. 1990. "Mothering Others' Children: The Experiences of Family Day Care Providers." In *Circles of Care: Work and Identity in Women's Lives*, edited by Emily K. Abel and Margaret K. Nelson, 210–32. Albany: State University of New York Press.

———. 2010. *Parenting out of Control: Anxious Parents in Uncertain Times*. New York: New York University Press.

———, Rosanna Hertz, and Wendy Kramer. 2013. "Making Sense of Donors and Donor Siblings: A Comparison of the Perceptions of Donor-Conceived Offspring in Lesbian-Parent and Heterosexual-Parent Families." In *Visions of the 21st Century Family: Transforming Structures and Identities*, edited by Patricia Neff Claster and Sampson Lee Blair, 1–42. Bingley, UK: Emerald Group Publishing.

Oakley, Ann. 1974. *Women's Work: The Housewife, Past and Present*. New York: Vintage.

Oliver, Kelly. 1989. "Marxism and Surrogacy." *Hypatia* 4 (3): 95–115.

Organization of Parents through Surrogacy. n.d. "Information about OPTS." Accessed July 16, 2015. http://www.opts.com/informat.htm.

Pande, Amrita. 2008. "Commercial Surrogate Mothering in India: Nine Months of Labor?" In *In Quest for Alternative Sociology*, edited by Kenji Kosaka and Masahiro Ogino, 71–87. Melbourne, Australia: Trans Pacific.

———. 2009. "'It May Be Her Eggs But It's My Blood': Surrogates and Everyday Forms of Kinship in India." *Qualitative Sociology* 32 (4): 379–405.

———. 2010a. "'At Least I Am Not Sleeping with Anyone': Resisting the Stigma of Commercial Surrogacy in India." Special issue on reproduction and mothering, *Feminist Studies* 36 (2): 292–312.

———. 2010b. "Commercial Surrogacy in India: Manufacturing a Perfect 'Mother-Worker.'" *Signs* 35 (4): 969–92.

———. 2014. *Wombs in Labor: Transnational Commercial Surrogacy in India*. New York: Columbia University Press.

Parente, Mary Ann A. 2004. "The Experience of Women Providing Gestational Surrogacy on Multiple Occasions." PhD diss., Massachusetts Institute of Technology.

Park, Kristin. 2002. "Stigma Management among the Voluntarily Childless." *Sociological Perspectives* 45 (1): 21–45.

Park, Lisa. 2005. *Consuming Citizenship: Children of Asian Immigrant Entrepreneurs*. Stanford, CA: Stanford University Press.

Parrenas, Rhacel. 2001. *Servants of Globalization: Women, Migration and Domestic Work.* Stanford, CA: Stanford University Press.

Pew Research Center. 2010. "The Decline of Marriage and the Rise of New Families." Accessed June 14, 2015. http://www.pewsocialtrends.org/2010/11/18/the-decline-of-marriage-and-rise-of-new-families/.

Poote, Aimee, and Olga van den Akker. 2009. "British Women's Attitudes to Surrogacy." *Human Reproduction* 24 (1): 139–45.

Purdy, Laura M. 1996. *Reproducing Persons: Issues in Feminist Bioethics.* Ithaca, NY: Cornell University Press.

Ragone, Helena. 1994. *Surrogate Motherhood: Conception in the Heart.* Boulder, CO: Westview.

———. 1999. "The Gift of Life: Surrogate Motherhood, Gamete Donation and Constructions of Altruism." In *Transformative Motherhood: On Giving and Getting in a Consumer Culture*, edited by Linda L. Layne, 65–88. New York: New York University Press.

Rao, Radhika. 2003. "Surrogacy Law in the United States: The Outcome of Ambivalence." In *Surrogate Motherhood: International Perspectives*, edited by Rachel Cook and Shelley Day Sclater with Felicity Kaganas, 23–34. Oxford: Hart.

Rapp, Rayna. 1997. "Constructing Amniocentesis: Maternal and Medical Discourses." In *Situated Lives: Gender and Culture in Everyday Life*, edited by Louise Lamphere, Helena Ragone, and Patricia Zavella, 128–41. New York: Routledge.

Reverby, Susan M. 1987. *Ordered to Care: The Dilemma of American Nursing 1850–1945.* New York: Cambridge University Press.

Roberts, Dorothy. 1997. *Killing the Black Body: Race, Reproduction, and the Meaning of Liberty.* New York: Pantheon.

———. 2002. *Shattered Bonds: The Color of Child Welfare.* New York: Basic.

Roberts, Elizabeth F. S. 1998. "Examining Surrogacy Discourses between Feminine Power and Exploitation." In *Small Wars: The Cultural Politics of Childhood*, edited by Nancy Scheper-Hughes and Carolyn Sargent, 93–110. Berkeley: University of California Press.

Romero, Mary. 1992. *Maid in the U.S.A.* New York: Routledge.

Rosenthal, Elisabeth. 2013. "American Way of Birth, Costliest in the World." *New York Times*, June 30. Accessed June 23, 2015. http://www.nytimes.com/2013/07/01/health/american-way-of-birth-costliest-in-the-world.html?hp&_r=3&.

Rothman, Barbara Katz. 1989. *Recreating Motherhood.* New Brunswick, NJ: Rutgers University Press.

———. 2011. "On Markens." *Sociological Forum* 26 (1): 201–5.

Rudrappa, Sharmila. 2010. "Outsourcing Labor: Transnational Surrogacy in India." *Research in the Sociology of Work* 20: 253–85.

———. 2012. "India's Reproductive Assembly Line." *Contexts* 11 (2): 22–27.

Russo, Nancy Felipe. 1976. "The Motherhood Mandate." *Journal of Social Issues* 32 (3): 143–53.

Saul, Stephanie. 2009. "Would-Be Parents Find Surrogate Agency Closed." *New York Times*, March 20.

Schneider, David M. 1968. *American Kinship: A Cultural Account.* Englewood Cliffs, NJ: Prentice-Hall.

Shanley, Mary Lyndon. 2001. *Making Babies, Making Families: What Matters Most in an Age of Reproductive Technologies, Surrogacy, Adoption, and Same-Sex and Unwed Parents.* Boston: Beacon.

Shetty, Priya. 2012. "India's Unregulated Surrogacy Industry." *Lancet* 380 (9854): 1633–34.

Smith, Dorothy. 1993. "The Standard North American Family: SNAF as an Ideological Code." *Journal of Family Issues* 14 (1): 50–65.

Society for Assisted Reproductive Technology. 2014. "Clinic Summary Report." Accessed June 11, 2015. https://www.sartcorsonline.com/rptCSR_PublicMultYear.aspx?ClinicPKID=0.

Solinger, Rickie. 2005. *Pregnancy and Power: A Short History of Reproductive Politics in America*. New York: New York University Press.

Spar, Debora L. 2006. *The Baby Business: How Money, Science, and Politics Drive the Commerce of Conception*. Boston: Harvard Business School Press.

Speier, Amy. 2011. "Brokers, Consumers, and the Internet: How North American Consumers Navigate Their Infertility Journeys." *Reproductive BioMedicine Online* 23 (5): 592–99.

State of Michigan Department of Human Services. n.d. "Adopting a Child in Michigan." Accessed July 16, 2015. http://www.michigan.gov/documents/dhs/DHS-PUB-0823_221566_7.pdf.

Sunderam, Saswati, Dmitry M. Kissin, Sara B. Crawford, Suzanne G. Folger, Denise J. Jamieson, and Wanda D. Barfied. 2014. "Assisted Reproductive Technology Surveillance—United States 2011." *Morbidity and Mortality Weekly Report*. Accessed July 13, 2015. http://www.cdc.gov/mmwr/preview/mmwrhtml/ss6310a1.htm.

Teman, Elly. 2008. "The Social Construction of Surrogacy Research: An Anthropological Critique of Psychosocial Scholarship on Surrogate Motherhood." *Social Science & Medicine* 67 (7): 1104–12.

———. 2010. *Birthing a Mother: The Surrogate Body and the Pregnant Self*. Berkeley: University of California Press.

Texas Family Code. n.d. "TEX FA. CODE ANN. § 160.754: Texas Statutes— Section 160.754: GESTATIONAL AGREEMENT AUTHORIZED." FindLaw. Accessed June 10, 2015. http://codes.lp.findlaw.com/txstatutes/FA/5/B/160/I/160.754.

Thompson, Charis. 2005. *Making Parents: The Ontological Choreography of Reproductive Technologies*. Cambridge, MA: MIT Press.

Titmuss, Richard M. 1997. *The Gift Relationship: From Human Blood to Social Policy*. Edited by Ann Oakley and John Ashton. Expanded and updated edition. New York: New Press.

Van den Akker, Olga. 2007. "Psychological Aspects of Surrogate Motherhood." *Human Reproduction* 13 (1): 53–66.

Van den Bos, Wouter, Eric van Dijk, and Eveline A. Crone. 2011. "Learning Whom to Trust in Repeated Social Interactions: A Developmental Perspective." *Group Processes & Intergroup Relations* 15 (2): 243–56.

Waldby, Katherine, and Robert Mitchell. 2006. *Tissue Economies: Blood, Organs, and Cell Lines in Late Capitalism*. Durham, NC: Duke University Press.

Weaver, Gillian, and A. Susan Williams. 1997. "A Mother's Gift: the Milk of Human Kindness." In Richard M. Titmuss, *The Gift Relationship: From Human Blood to Social Policy*, edited by Ann Oakley and John Ashton, 319–32. Expanded and updated edition. New York: New Press.

Wegar, Katarina. 1997. *Adoption, Identity, and Kinship: The Debate over Sealed Birth Records*. New Haven, CT: Yale University Press.

Weiss, Gregory L. 1992. "Public Attitudes about Surrogate Motherhood." *Michigan Sociological Review* 6: 15–27.

Weston, Kath. 1997. *Families We Choose: Lesbians, Gays, Kinship*. New York: Columbia University Press.

"Who's Who in the Fight for Baby M." 1987. *New York Times*, April 1.

Yngvesson, Barbara. 2004. "Going 'Home': Adoption, Exclusive Belongings, and the Mythology of Roots." In *Consuming Motherhood*, edited by Janelle S. Taylor, Linda L. Layne, and Danielle F. Wozniak, 168–86. New Brunswick, NJ: Rutgers University Press.

Zarembo, Alan. 2011. "Scam Targeted Surrogates as Well as Couples." *Los Angeles Times*, August 13. Accessed June 12, 2015. http://articles.latimes.com/2011/aug/13/local/la-me-baby-ring-20110814.

Zelizer, Viviana. 1985. *Pricing the Priceless Child: The Changing Social Values of Children*. Princeton, NJ: Princeton University Press.

———. 2005. *The Purchase of Intimacy*. Princeton, NJ: Princeton University Press.

Zweig, Michael. 2000. *The Working Class Majority: America's Best Kept Secret*. Ithaca, NY: ILR Press.

Index

About the Author

HEATHER JACOBSON is an associate professor of sociology at the University of Texas at Arlington and the author of *Culture Keeping: White Mothers, International Adoption, and the Negotiation of Family Difference.*